CUPPING THERAPY

THE PRACTICAL GUIDE TO GETTING STARTED WITH THE HEALING PRACTICE

MICHAEL L. ZHANG

A D

© Copyright 2020 - All rights reserved Admore Publishing

ISBN: 978-3-96772-009-9 (Paperback)

The content contained within this book may not be reproduced, duplicated or transmitted without direct written permission from the author or the publisher.

Under no circumstances will any blame or legal responsibility be held against the publisher, or author, for any damages, reparation, or monetary loss due to the information contained within this book. Either directly or indirectly.

The cover for this work was created with the help of an image from "Depositphotos".

The Icons used in this work were designed by:

- Good Ware from www.flaticon.com
- Freepik from www.flaticon.com
- Macrovector from www.freepik.com
- rawpixel.com from www.freepik.com

Legal Notice:

This book is copyright protected. This book is only for personal use. You cannot amend, distribute, sell, use, quote or paraphrase any part, or the content within this book, without the consent of the author or publisher.

Please note the information contained within this document is for educational and entertainment purposes only. All effort has been executed to present accurate, up to date, and reliable, complete information. No warranties of any kind are declared or implied. Readers acknowledge that the author is not engaging in the rendering of legal, financial, medical or professional advice. The content within this book has been derived from various sources. Please consult a licensed professional before attempting any techniques outlined in this book.

By reading this document, the reader agrees that under no circumstances is the author responsible for any losses, direct or indirect, which are incurred as a result of the use of information contained within this document, including, but not limited to, — errors, omissions, or inaccuracies.

www.publishing.admore-marketing.com

Disclaimer

This book is a collection of information from the top experts in cupping therapy. All details have been carefully researched and selected but are for informational purposes only. It is not intended to be interpreted as professional medical advice or replace consultation with health care professionals.

Speak to your trusted healthcare professional prior to undergoing any medical procedures, or taking any nutritional supplements. Reactions and results vary from each individual as there are differences in health conditions.

If you have any underlying health conditions, consult with an appropriately licensed healthcare professional before considering any guidance from this book.

CONTENTS

Foreword	vii
1. Introduction	1
2. History	7
3. Benefits of Cupping	13
4. What to Consider Before Starting	19
5. Home vs Clinic	27
6. Types of Cups	33
7. Methods of Cupping	43
8. Placements for Treatments - Location Pains	59
9. Placements for Treatments - Illnesses & Issues	111
10. Placements for Treatments - Beauty	131
11. After Therapy	141
Thank you!	149
Sources & References	151

FOREWORD

> "The greatest medicine of all is to teach people how not to need it." - *Hippocrates*

... Thank you to Sandra for inspiring me. Dedicated to my two cats Snickers & Snackers.

Chapter 1

INTRODUCTION

WHAT IS CUPPING?

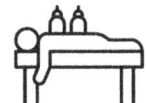

Cupping...

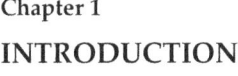ost of us are introduced to this unique therapy after noticing someone with large round "hickey" like marks on their skin. You may have noticed markings on athletes or celebrities on TV that sparked your curiosity. It may even have been recommended to you by a friend or professional practitioner. Most everyone wonders and asks...

... Why would anyone want to go through this process?

There are many reasons, as the practice helps deal with pain, blood flow, inflammation, and general well-being. Some athletes compare it to receiving a deep-tissue massage. The procedure is painless and is described by many as a soothing and relaxing experience. Although many use the therapy for pain relief and for helping with recovery, it is also a popular preventative treatment. Some undergo the procedure to help with flow and the releasing of tension. The marks left behind on the skin are temporary and last about 3 to 7 days on average.

Although it may seem like a new, trendy health rage, the truth is, the therapy has been around for a long time.

Cupping is an ancient form of alternative medicine that has been used for thousands of years. The origin of the therapy is still uncertain, however, it dates back to the ancient Egyptian, Middle Eastern, and Chinese cultures.

Cupping has greatly evolved from its ancient beginnings with more advanced tools and continues to be a popular way for individuals to heal in a natural way. Although the process looks intricate, the science behind the therapy is relatively simple. It is all based on blood flow. In today's fast-paced world is is common to reach for pills, be it anti-inflammatories, pain relievers, or any other quick fix medications. Cupping therapy is effective as it utilizes your body's natural way of healing. An expert simply targets specific areas that need to recover.

"Blood flow is the body's way of naturally healing," explains Houman Danesh, M.D. an Associate Professor at Mount Sinai Hospital who specializes in pain management and rehabilitation & physical medicine. Dr. Houman often combines different pain therapies with cupping to help his patients heal and recover.

"Increased blood flow can be beneficial to jumpstart or restart a blunted healing response." *Houman Danesh, M.D.*

Cupping allows us to guide the body into starting an inflammatory response. This organizes antibodies to a specific area on the body to try to heal it. For individuals like athletes, the increased blood flow helps repair muscle fibers after competitions or workouts. For others with pain-based conditions, cupping therapy can be used to help with area specific ailments like shoulder pain, lower back pain, fibromyalgia, and plantar fasciitis.

. . .

How it Works

The therapy is started by placing special suction cups on specific areas of a patient's body. The areas where the cups are placed depend on what needs to be treated. The cups themselves also vary. We will explore the different kinds of cups used in Chapter 6, however, most commonly glass, plastic, or silicone cups are used. The suction process also varies, although it is most commonly achieved by either heating the air inside of a cup or by using an air pump to suction out the air.

This allows for an anti-gravitational pull to take place and for the skin tissue to be pulled outwards rather than pushed inwards. It can be considered the opposite of a traditional massage. This outward pull promotes blood flow to specific areas and treatments are often times combined with massages to really get things flowing. This allows the body to naturally heal and recover.

Cupping therapy draws many similarities to acupuncture. Both of the therapies are key components of traditional Chinese medicine. In acupuncture *Qi (chi)* is drawn to specific areas that are blocked or poorly circulating. Similarly, with cupping the suction effect is also positioned in a specific area and draws blood flow. Some practitioners even combine acupuncture and cupping to provide further benefits to their patients.

. . .

Methods

There are several techniques when it comes this practice. We will take a deep dive into the different methods practitioners use in Chapter 7, however, there are two main forms of the therapy.

<u>Dry cupping and wet cupping.</u>

In simple terms, dry cupping involves no incision into the skin and wet cupping pertains to an expert making light incisions into the skin. In wet cupping therapy, impure blood and toxins are pulled out of the body. As mentioned above, we will look into more of the methods used in Chapter 7. While we will cover various techniques and ideologies of cupping the main applications throughout this book are for dry cupping techniques.

This was a small look into one of the few practices that has survived thousands of years to still being prevalent today. People all over the world use the therapy to stop pain, treat injuries, and promote their overall health and wellbeing. In this book we will look at everything from the history of cupping to the equipment necessary, and how to go about using the therapy to combat specific ailments. We consider the best practices and where to place cups for different treatments. We will also cover various safety measures and what to consider after a session.

Chapter 2

HISTORY

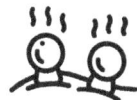

This holistic treatment method has been around for centuries. The therapy has roots in a variety of countries and cultures which makes the true origin difficult to determine. Some experts believe that the concept of cupping was already being used by prehistoric humans. It is instinctual for humans to attempt to suck blood out from a wound or bite. In essence, that is already a form of cupping.

When the practice truly started, cupping looked very different. The cups used for the therapy were nothing like what we have available to us today. They were made out of distinct items like animal horns, bamboo, shells, and clay. With these tools, practitioners would manually suck air out of the tips of the objects.

As the treatment gained popularity through success, it was introduced to a variety of ancient cultures.

Earliest Signs

It continues to be a controversial topic, however, the earliest use of the practice dates back to one of the oldest medical textbooks. The *Ebers Papyrus*. It was written around 1550 BC, and documents how the Egyptians used cupping to heal a variety of illnesses. It described how people of the Sahara used hollowed animal horns as cups to drain toxins and impurities out of the ill. Cupping was used to help heal everything from different pains to illnesses like fever.

Over a thousand years after the Egyptians, the art of treatment was passed on to ancient Greeks. The famous physicians Hippocrates and Galen were strong advocates practice. They would use cupping to treat various structural problems along with internal diseases. The cups of this time had evolved from animal horns to being made out of bronze.

China

Cupping is one of the staples of traditional Chinese medicine. Chinese medical traditions are based on and

Cupping Therapy

have evolved for over 3,500 years of practice. Cupping is one of the therapies that has been there from the beginning and remains highly prevalent in hospitals today.

Just as in Egypt, the first cups used were hollowed out cattle horns. These then evolved into bamboo cups that were boiled in water or placed under a flame to be able to suck a patient's skin. Initially, cupping was only used to draw out blood and impurities as an additional method in traditional Chinese surgery. Overtime, it was found that cupping was useful in treating other diseases and therapeutic methods evolved.

In China the earliest found records which describe the process of cupping is an ancient book written on silk called the *Bo Shu* (Estimated time period between 206 BC - 210 AD). After the Bo Shu, a variety of other ancient texts discuss the practice and its uses for successful treatments.

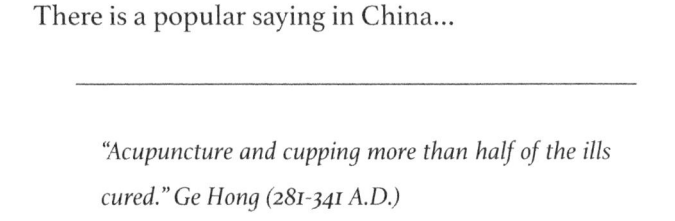

There is a popular saying in China...

"Acupuncture and cupping more than half of the ills cured." Ge Hong (281-341 A.D.)

Over thousands of years the experience of Chinese

practitioners has evolved and clinical applications of cupping have increased. Now Chinese medicine cupping is used to treat skin conditions, chronic cough, asthma, indigestion issues, and even arthritic symptoms.

Although there are electronic suction cups available, in China the traditional tools are still often used. Bamboo and horns are a rare sighting, however, practitioners continue to use the traditional glass cups. Especially in more rural areas where more modern western medicine is not as readily available the practice is used to help many patients.

Other Cultures and Areas

Over time, the therapy found its way throughout the Middle East, Asia, and finally Europe. In the Middle East several countries use the therapy. In Arabic, cupping is known as *Hijama*. The founder of Islam, Muhammad, mentioned cupping often throughout his teachings and writings. There are many Islamic medical texts that describe many of the best practices of the therapy.

In the 19th and early 20th centuries, cupping was common practice throughout Europe. It was regularly used for treating a variety of conditions like ingestion, muscular problems, colds, chest pains, and the flu. European and American doctors widely used cupping in practice until the late 1800's.

As different areas of western modern medicine advanced, cupping began to fall out of practice. It was largely due to lack of understanding and interest as different, more modern medical advances grew. Today a variety of drugs, machines, and new technology flood the market, however there is an ever increasing interest in cupping once again. With top athletes and celebrities like Michael Phelps, Stephen Curry, Natalie Coughlin, Victoria Beckham, Justin Bieber, and Jenifer Aniston often undergoing the procedure, the therapy is experiencing a resurgence of interest. There are many healthcare professionals that offer cupping and promote the therapy for healing.

Chapter 3
BENEFITS OF CUPPING

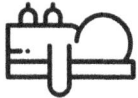

Cupping allows for blood to flow to targeted areas on the body. It is said that this increase in blood circulation promotes pain relief, general healing, and the removal of toxins. Through stretching and contracting the skin, blood flows and jump-starts healing. Reid Blackwelder, M.D., refers to it as "sterile inflammation". The cupping process pulls blood from a patient's vessels into their tissue. This mobilizes antibodies to an area which attempt to heal any issues there. It should be noted that this may be the reason why the therapy is used to treat location based pains.

As blood is transferred to the area underneath each individual cup, all the local cells can repair faster. The bruising marks often observed on individuals who just completed a cupping session are the display of blood being drawn to the area. So much blood is circulating specific points that capillaries are overrun and leave the bruising marks. In Kenneth Choi's (R.Ac & R.TCMP) book, *Cupping Therapy for Muscles and Joints,* he describes the effect of these ruptures having the same benefits as autohemotherapy, only through a less invasive procedure. In autohemotherapy blood is drawn out of a patient and then re-injected. This is believed to help fight disease and boost the immune system.

Throughout this chapter we will explore the various benefits cupping therapy is said to have.

Treatments of Pain & Injury

Cupping has been used for years to help with a variety of treatments, be it pains or injuries. Pain in the neck, back, shoulders, and knees can all be relieved through the influx of blood flow and stimulation of specific points. Much like in acupuncture, which some specialists use in combination with cupping therapy, throughout a session endorphins, cortisol, and serotonin are released. These chemicals are produced naturally by the body to help us cope with pain or stress. Often they are referred to as "feel-good" chemicals as they make us feel happy and are natural pain relievers. The therapy has the ability to increase the pain threshold in the area. Cupping is said to stimulate specific nerve fibers that both reduce pain and block pain messages from reaching the brain.

Muscle Stiffness

Several top athletes have used cupping to speed up recovery from injury and muscle stiffness. Heavy workouts place a lot of stress on muscles which cause them to tighten and tear. Cupping therapy allows muscles to loosen and recover faster, and the individual to feel relief. Cupping will lift fascia, which is connective tissue underneath the skin that attaches, stabilizes, encloses, and separates muscles and other internal organs. Through lifting this connective tissue, muscles can loosen and recover more easily.

Recovery

A few symptoms that many deal with are muscle aches, nausea, and stomach pains. This can be because of a buildup of lactic acid. Lactic acid builds up in muscles and cupping therapy allows for blood to flush out these toxic buildups. The increased blood flow the therapy provides helps repair muscle fibers and flush out any unwanted impurities.

. . .

Relaxation

The therapy can help be a relaxing force in a patient's life. Not only are "feel-good" chemicals released into your bloodstream through the process, it is often also referred to being similar to a deep-tissue massage. After placing the cups on a patient, some practitioners continue the therapy by sliding the cups along an area. This process is called "walking cups" or moving cupping. It is usually performed on a patient's back after it has been properly lubricated with natural oils encouraging relaxation. The therapy is generally completed in a comforting environment as a patient should feel comfortable and pain free at all times.

Beauty

Modern cupping has evolved from strictly a healing therapy to being used for cosmetic purposes. As blood flow is improved, and capillaries are expanded, skin is firmed and toned. Cupping therapy is able to boost skin health and can be used to combat cellulite, acne, and different skin inflammations. Cellulite and acne are caused by waste and dirt that is trapped just underneath the skin. Cupping increases blood circulation in these problem areas and allows your body to flush out problematic wastes and toxins. The results will leave a patient with smoother and firmer skin.

Alternative Benefits

Traditional Chinese medicine along with other cultures believe that cupping improves *Qi* (Chi). Qi is free flowing vital energy that circulates through the world and in our bodies. If Qi is interrupted or blocked an individual will feel pain or aches because there is an imbalance in the body.

Energy Flow

Cupping therapy assists energy flow within the body. Practitioners will target specific parts of the body to help clear blockages or stagnant areas. After sessions, Qi or vital energy can flow freely again. Negative energy along with other impurities are removed. Traditional Chinese medicine believes that cupping enhances not only the physical well-being of a patient, but also the emotional well-being.

Detoxification

In traditional Chinese medicine it is believed that cupping brings *defensive Qi* to blocked or affected areas.

The modern medical explanation of defensive Qi can be considered white blood cells. These are cells of the immune system that help protect the body against all impurities. The job of white blood cells is to destroy harmful substances. Cupping directs white blood cells to specific areas, and this assists detoxification. The therapy helps clear blockages and release contaminants.

Chapter 4

WHAT TO CONSIDER BEFORE STARTING

Although cupping has numerous benefits for many, there are some things to consider before potentially starting with the practice. There may be different reasons you are considering taking part in the therapy, however, it is best to look at possible side effects. Some simply should not take part in the practice. In the following section we will explore things to be aware of along with possible side effects. If you are unsure regarding any medical conditions, please discuss them with a doctor or field expert.

Possible Side Effects

The round markings that a cupping leaves behind is

well known. While it is a temporary side effect of the practice, it is something to be aware of. The markings disappear after a couple of days or slightly after a week. The severity of these markings is dependent on how strong the suction is within each cup. An experienced practitioner will be able to determine what suction strength is appropriate. Many of the side effects listed below can easily be avoided and only occur with unprepared practitioners. Cupping therapy may cause the following side effects:

Bruises

As stated above, these are normal, painless marks that remain after a session. It is, however, important that the practitioner follows standard infection control practices and safety precautions. This protects bruises from infections and other unwanted ailments.

Skin Infections

Skin infections are rare in the practice however can happen when the treatment is completed unprofessionally. A practitioner should clean and disinfect the areas they will work on before cupping and post cupping. Furthermore, all utilized tools should either be new for every patient or properly disinfected.

Soreness & Discomfort

A proper cupping session is a relaxing experience. One should feel no discomfort and leave the practice feeling relieved from pains or stresses. As with all the potential side effects of the practice, they pertain to the practitioner. A patient should voice their concerns immediately if they feel uncomfortable or in pain at any time during a session. If suction within a cup is too strong, it may place too much stress on an individual. This has no place in the therapy and creates the potential of doing more harm than good for a patient.

Burns

There are a variety of methods used to create suction within cups for the therapy. The two most common ways are by either manually removing air from a cup with a hand pump, or with heat. Heat is a more traditional way of creating suction within a cup. A practitioner will heat the inside of a cup with a flame which removes oxygen and then quickly place the cup on a patient's body. The lack of oxygen creates a vacuum, and this allows the cup to attach to a patient's skin. Unprofessional or inexperienced practitioners may not properly dose a flame and overly heat cups. This is highly hazardous for a patient as it risks burns.

Most of these side effects can be prevented and demonstrate the importance of dealing with proper healthcare professionals. Unfortunately, there is no regulatory body for cupping therapy however, there are a wide range of expert practitioners in the following fields:

- Medical Doctors
- Physiotherapists
- Chiropractors
- TCM (Traditional Chinese Medicine) Practitioners
- Acupuncturists
- Massage therapists

Cupping Therapy is not for...

Cupping helps many increase blood circulation, relieve pain, remove toxins and much more. The therapy does however have its limits, and should not be used by everyone. There isn't tremendous stress placed on the body but individuals of a certain age, or with specific ailments will unfortunately need different solutions. Cupping therapy is not suitable for individuals:

With blood thinning medication

As the practice increases blood circulation, those taking blood thinners risk placing too much stress on their capillaries. Those with other blood related disorders like thrombocytopenia should also avoid cupping.

With skin conditions

Cupping should not be performed on those who have inflamed skin and a variety of skin conditions like psoriasis, vitiligo, and rosacea. Cupping can improve skin conditions, however, should not be applied directly to skin that is broken, irritated, or inflamed. Those with highly sensitive skin, skin allergies, and rashes are not suitable patients.

Who are pregnant

Pregnant women should avoid the practice.

That are too young or old

It is recommended that patients are at least 18 years old. Older candidates need to be evaluated on a case-by-case basis. Seniors of a certain age will no longer be able to recover from the potential bruising that occurs during the therapy.

With severe health conditions

Individuals with certain health conditions should not get started with the therapy. Organ failure, heart diseases, cancer, edema, hemophilia, diabetes, broken bones, and fibromyalgia are all examples of conditions that are inappropriate for cupping therapy. Furthermore, those with medical implants such as pacemakers, computer implants, and insulin pumps should avoid the practice.

Cupping is said to be an excellent way to promote circulation and has tremendous health benefits. It is however important to be aware of all the potential side effects, along with if the therapy is appropriate for a specific situation. It is essential to deal with experienced and professional practician. Many of the side effects are avoided when dealing with an expert. Also, a proper practician will use a combination of conventional treatment along with cupping therapy. Researches stress that cupping should be used as an alternative or complementary treatment.

Chapter 5
HOME VS CLINIC

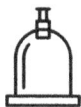

There are several reasons someone may look to get started with the practice. Health, beauty, or spiritual reasons are all viable aims just to name a few. Many question, however, is the practice something safe to do by themselves, or is it something that should be left to the professionals? At-home cupping therapy kits are more easily available than ever. In the following chapter, we will consider whether the practice is manageable at home, or if one should consider visiting a professional.

Professional Practitioners

Throughout Chapter 4 we explored the possible side

effects of the practice. When the therapy is completed correctly, it allows for the improved circulation and blood flow, leading to enhanced nerve function. Unfortunately, if the practice is completed incorrectly, it can lead to a number of complications like nerve damage, burning, blistering, and more.

Generally it is recommended to have the procedure completed by a professional. Technically, cupping is a medical procedure. Modern tools for the therapy are readily available and make the process more manageable from home. However, if you feel uncertain or uncomfortable, it is best to see a professional.

Cupping is often used as an alternative or complementary treatment. This demonstrates how professionals handle any health complications. They discuss the options available to work on ailments directly with patients. Often those who start with cupping therapy with a practitioner decide to continue with the practice at home. A professional will have already guided them through their first sessions and then they are comfortable continuing by themselves.

At Home

Traditionally, even modern cupping required glass cups along with a flame. This made the practice hazardous and not particularly beginner friendly. Today, a variety of cups are available, made out of materials like plastic and silicone. Also, suction has evolved from strictly requiring a flame to suction pumps. This makes the treatments at home much safer and far more accessible.

It is important to realize, however, that many of the side effects mentioned in Chapter 4 should still be concerns for those looking to take the practice home. Not developing a deep understanding of the practice can lead to serious conditions. Some may also face the issue that more affordable at-home products may not yield the same results as visiting a professional.

At-home kits generally feature cups made out of plastic or silicone. While cups made out of these materials may give excellent results, there will be some options that do not measure up to professional quality equipment. The kits can be great for beginners and help ensure a safe practice, however, they may not ensure the proper amount of suction required. This can lead to poor results. In the following section we will explore some details to be aware of for using the practice at home:

Cleanliness

While dry cupping is non-invasive, it remains a medical procedure. The area that is worked on will need to be cleaned and disinfected before and after the therapy. The area must be dry and clean. Some practitioners include essential oils in a therapy session. It is common for to add oils before positioning the cups or post-treatment to promote healing and further blood flow. Some patients with excessive body hair may choose to shave the areas to be treated. The suction may be uncomfortable if the areas have several hair follicles.

Proper Placement

It is important to know where to place cups. Some appropriate areas for proper cup placement are displayed in Chapters 8 through 10.

Some general guidelines for the practice are to position cups on fleshy areas of the body. This includes the back, legs, arms, and stomach. For treating pain or for general recovery, those are excellent points. It is best to not place cups on areas where one can feel a pulse. Areas with ulcers, vein thrombosis, or arteries should be steered clear of.

If using the therapy to treat a specific condition, it is best to have a professional first determine the appropriate points. Once the points are determined, and a patient feels comfortable, then it is recommended to commence treatment at home.

Appropriate Equipment

The therapy is only effective with the appropriate equipment. Once this is confirmed is is also fundamental to properly store and care for the equipment. The cups must be cleaned and cared for accordingly or a patient risks infections and other unwanted side effects. Other potential tools such as pumps, rubbing alcohol, or tubes must be stored and cared for properly as well.

While it is possible to follow the guidelines that come with an at-home cupping therapy kit and successfully complete a practice, it does come with potential risks. It is better to be introduced to the practice by a professional that can guide one along properly. Stephanie Tyiska, a NCCAOM-certified acupuncturist and Chinese herbal medicine practitioner explains that "It's always best to spend the money and have a treatment with a specialist first so you've experienced the processes and results on your skin".

It is recommended to experience some expert hands-on advice before experimenting with the therapy. A patient will feel appropriate levels of suction and experience first hands the wonders of the therapy.

Chapter 6
TYPES OF CUPS

There are a variety of cups used in cupping therapy. The "cups" evolved greatly, starting out as animal horns and evolving to pots, then glass, and eventually the modern sets we have available today. Suction methods have also undergone a transformation. From manual suction, to a flame, to a variety of methods used today.

Throughout this chapter we will explore different cupping sets along with suction methods. Each cup has their own applications, and positives and negatives. There are a variety techniques when it comes to cupping and different cups will be appropriate for a specific technique. First, we will look at some of the more traditional cups that are sometimes still used today, and then we will examine more modern appliances.

Pottery

Practitioners rarely use these types of cups for cupping therapy. There are much more effective and safer solutions available today, however some prefer to use traditional tools. The cups or jars are made out of clay and shaped into the appropriate form and size. The mouth of the cup is of a smaller circumference and the body is much larger. The bottom of the clay pot is flat. Once the cup is shaped, it gets hardened through heat and the cup is ready for the therapy.

Practitioners using these cups can get a lot of suction out of them. They have a very strong suction strength that is believed to enhance energy within the body. These cups are very fragile, however, and heavy. This makes them difficult for a practitioner to handle and so are no longer considered appropriate for the therapy. It is also difficult to view suction strength as one cannot monitor the situation inside of a cup. This can be dangerous as patients risk blistering or burning their skin.

Bamboo

Cups made of bamboo were mostly used in China. Throughout some parts of China, along with some traditional Chinese medicine practitioners, the use of bamboo cups is still prevalent. A cupping technique, *herbal cupping,* is often practiced with bamboo cups. The technique allows for bamboo to absorb specific herbs that promote healing. More information on herbal cupping can be found in Chapter 7.

Bamboo cups were often used for the therapy as it is an easily available material. It is also very durable and is perfect for herbal cupping techniques. The cups are relatively lightweight, strong enough to survive a drop, and can be stored easily. There are, however, some issues with using bamboo cups. Just as with pottery cups, a practitioner cannot accurately monitor the suction strength on a patient. The bamboo cups are not transparent, and so there is no way to determine suction. Also, the cups are difficult to clean. Bamboo wood is lightly porous which makes it excellent for herbal cupping but difficult to clean. Older cups, or cups that were not properly cared for also risk splintering. This can be highly discomforting to patients and may tear skin.

Glass

Glass cups have transitioned beautifully from traditional to modern methods of cupping. Glass cups have been used for centuries, and they continue to be some of the most widely used cups today. There are a variety of techniques used in cupping therapy. Glass cups can be used for all techniques except one; herbal cupping. The material is perfect for all other methods used in the practice.

Glass cups are easily available in different shapes and sizes which allow them to be used in a variety of places on a patient's body. Glass is also very easy to clean and sterilize. Patients won't risk infections as the materials will be clean. The material is also transparent, which allows a practitioner to properly monitor suction strength. A practitioner can be sure suction is exactly where it needs to be. The only negative aspect of glass cups is fragility. There is no real risk of a cup cracking or breaking because of strong suction, however, an accidental drop will likely break a cup.

Traditional glass cups are shaped in a rounded form. A practitioner uses a flame to remove the air from inside a class and then quickly place the cup on a patient. The lack or oxygen in the cup allows for a vacuum effect to take place, and the cup to stick on a patient. This is the traditional method used, and it requires an experienced practitioner. The combinations of an open flame, suction strength, and glass is difficult to master without appropriate training.

Modern glass cups include a nozzle at the top. The nozzle allows a practitioner to attach a manual pump and determine suction strength without having to use a flame. These improvements have made the practice safer, as there are fewer risks involved. Other modern glass cups include a vacuum twist-top nozzle, which also allows a practitioner to manually add suction to a cup.

Plastic

Plastic is a common material used for modern cups. They are not often used in clinics as practitioners there will likely prefer medical grade glass cups instead. For individual or at home use, plastic cupping sets perform very well. They can provide great suction control, and they are durable. The material will survive accidental drops, and since the cups are transparent, a practitioner will be able to carefully monitor suction.

Similar as modern glass cups, there are two main ways to gain suction in a plastic cup. There are twist-tops and manual pumps. Later on in the chapter we will look deeper into the different suction methods available.

Silicone

Silicone cups are highly durable, as they can bend and twist into practically any direction or form. Just like plastic cups, silicone cups are a popular at-home cupping set solution. Strong cleaning or disinfecting products can damage silicone. This makes the material unsuitable for clinical use. For at home use, however, cupping sets made of silicone are optimal. The cups are easy to apply by pushing downward against skin. This releases air out of the cup and allows the cup to stick. Suction is easily determined by either pushing out more or less air.

A weakness of silicone cups is that suction strength will not be as high as the other cups mentioned before. Silicone is a very forgiving material so it will not remain as rigid as the other materials like glass or plastic. It is a great beginners set, that is light to transport and easy to use. These sets are available in a variety of sizes to assist treatment of a variety of ailments in different areas of the body.

Suction

Suction is one of the most crucial aspect of the therapy. It is what makes the healing practice unique. Cupping is the only process that allows for any anti-gravitational pulls on a patient's body. Massages are an excellent way of releasing tension in muscles, however, it only offers downward compression. Cupping therapy works by using negative pressure to improve blood flow, inflammation, range of motion, and much more. The main element involved in this is *suction*.

So how is this suction created?

There are 4 common ways practitioners create suction within cups.

Flame

The traditional way of gaining suction in a cup is through the help of a flame. Although it is an older technique, it is still used today as it proves to be highly effective. The science behind the technique is simple. Fire uses oxygen to burn. If the oxygen within a cup is removed, it will create a vacuum effect and this suction will allow the cup to remain attached to skin. Thus, if a flame enters a cup, it will use all the oxygen inside of it causing the vacuum effect. If a cup is then quickly placed on skin, it will remain attached.

At a clinic, a practitioner will soak a cotton ball in 95% alcohol. The soaked cotton ball is then removed from the alcohol with pincers and carefully lit on fire. The practitioner will then stick the cotton ball into a glass cup for about a second. Then quickly remove it, and in the same motion place the cup on the area to be treated. The process is fast because air will enter the cup again if a practitioner waits too long.

This suction method requires appropriate training and practice. Any situation with an open flame commands caution. At a proper clinic with a qualified practitioner, the technique is safe and effective. A patient should not feel much of the heat on their back, only a soothing warm effect. A properly qualified practitioner will make their patients feel comfortable at all times and ensure that therapy is completed in a professional manner.

Manual Pump

Suction through the help of a manual pump is a more modern technique used by practitioners. It requires no flame or heat that can potentially burn a patient. The method is usually applied to either special glass or plastic cups. The cups will include a nozzle that can attach to a manual pump.

A practitioner will attach a hand pump with tubing to the end of a cups nozzle. Once a practitioner has placed the cup on the area that is going to be treated, the hand pump can be used to manually create suction. It varies pump to pump, however, half a pump to one pump will be enough to create light suction. One to two pumps will create medium suction, and above this will create strong suction.

This suction method is suitable for most cupping techniques. It comes down to what material the cups are made out of, for example, glass versus plastic. The suction method is more beginner friendly than using a flame. A practitioner can assess suction strength easily, and can quickly apply more by pumping or lightly release tension by letting some air enter a cup.

Twist

Another modern technique to gain suction within a cup utilizes a twist function. This technique requires special cups that have a twisting rotor. These cups are often made of plastic but can also be found in glass form. The twist tops are almost always made out of plastic.

Cups using this technique gain suction by increasing and decreasing the amount of space inside of a cup. Once a practitioner places a cup on a patient, the inside of the cup becomes air tight. Then similarly to a screwdriver, if the top of the cup's rotor is twisted upwards (in most cases to the left) the space inside the cup gets increased. Since the cup is airtight, the movement will create suction and a patient's skin is drawn upwards.

This technique simplifies the cupping process. The suction strength can easily be monitored and adjusted. Depending on the material of the cups (plastic, or glass) it can be appropriately used for a variety of cupping methods.

Push/Squeeze

Suction through squeezing or pushing is reserved only for silicone cupping sets. Silicone is flexible and allows itself to be compressed. This is a great option for beginners as the material is very forgiving and gaining suction is easy to achieve. Silicone is also durable and will survive accidental drops.

A practitioner can create suction by placing the cup on the desired location and simply pushing downward. The further down the cup is pushed the greater the suction will be. This suction technique is great for minor aches or pains and is also excellent for skin care applications. It is believed to be a great solution for battling cellulite and wrinkles.

Chapter 7
METHODS OF CUPPING

There are several cupping therapy techniques practitioners use to produce the most benefits for their patients. Although many methods all produce a similar baseline of benefits, different applications are used for different purposes. It can be noted that some techniques will require different tools, or more specifically, cups and suctioning methods. We explored the different cups used throughout the therapy in more detail in Chapter 6.

Before we look into the different techniques practitioners use, we will observe the different suction strengths, and the different effects these have on the practice. These different suction strengths can be combined with all the different techniques practitioners use.

Suction Strength

Weak:

Weak suction allows for the most gentle version of the therapy. A patient's skin is pulled upwards as lightly as possible while still remaining attached to a cup. This version of the practice is great for weaker patients (older or younger individuals) who need to improve organ function and further nourish the body.

This strength will not leave any strong bruise marks except on patients with highly sensitive skin. There may be some light discoloration however that will likely fade within an hour.

It is said that this suction strength allows the body to best re-energize. It will not help get rid of toxins as the pull is not strong enough. Weak suction still assists energy and blood flow as a practitioner can still bring nourishment to weaker areas.

How To:

Weak suction may seem easy to achieve, however it requires some practice. The trick is to get as light of a suction as possible inside a cup that is strong enough to maintain steady on a patient's body. Depending on how suction is achieved in a cup (pump/twist/push/heat), create as light a suction as possible. It usually requires minimum effort.

A great aspect of the practice is that it is simple to lighten the suction level within a cup. It is possible to allow some air into a cup and release some tension. This is achieved by lightly pressing down on the skin next to a cup with one hand while carefully lifting up the side of the cup with the other hand. This allows some air to enter the cup and releases some of the tension. This process can be completed with any cup type.

Medium:

A medium level of suction is simply a level above light suction. It is the level that is most often used throughout the therapy. Due to the stronger pull, it is normal for darker marks or bruising to occur. The negative pressure is commonly used to help drain excess fluids and toxins, bring blood flow to stagnant skin and muscles, loosen adhesions, and stimulate the peripheral nervous system.

This level of suction can potentially still be used on weaker patients, however, a practitioner will need to carefully assess the situation. The patient will require less time, along with fewer cups.

How To:

Medium suction will require approximately double the amount of suction compared to light suction. A practitioner should carefully monitor the suction level and whereas the skin on a patient with light cupping should only lightly appear elevated, with medium cupping it should appear clearly lifted.

As with light suction, it is possible to ease tension on the skin by manually allowing some air to enter a cup. This reduces suction and eases pressure on an area.

Strong:

Strong suction allows for the severest suction strength in the practice. It is most commonly used to help drain out toxins, lift connective tissue, and improving blood flow.

This level of suction will leave some bruise marks that

can take some days or weeks to remove. It will take the body longest to recover from a session that involves strong suction.

How To:

Strong suction is the most powerful suction level possible in the practice, while remaining helpful and pain-free for a patient. It is crucial for a practitioner to monitor the cups at this level of suction and ensure that a patient is comfortable and remains pain free at all times. The skin inside a cup at this suction level will be lifted up to an inch high. A practitioner should follow this carefully and make sure not to increase pressure above this.

Just as with all the other suction levels, it is possible to release tension by allowing some air to enter a cup. It is vital to continue to check on the cups at this pressure as a patient's skin risks blistering.

Techniques

Dry Cupping

Dry cupping describes a basic form of the therapy that

also happens to be one that is used most often. A practitioner will effectively apply glass, plastic, silicone, or bamboo cups to a patient's skin. The cups will remain still on the skin for 10 to 30 minutes depending on suction strength and what needs to be treated.

Throughout dry cupping, cups are placed over several areas to lift soft tissue and create an upward pull or stretch effect. The process eases muscle tension, along with any associated pain. Dry cupping can be completed with any of the cup types available, which we described in Chapter 6.

What differentiates "dry" cupping from other techniques is that the cups are left in a static position. There are no incisions made in a patients skin that a practitioner will need to constantly monitor. A practitioner also does not need to remain active and move the cups around. As cupping is often prescribed as a complementary treatment, a practitioner can utilise the therapy to aid treatment more efficiently. For instance, cups can be placed in one area to pre-reduce muscle tension and increase blood flow, as another area is being treated manually. This speeds up recovery and allows for a combination of healing practices.

Wet Cupping

Cupping Therapy

Wet cupping is a technique that is more commonly used in Islamic cultures and is less prevalent in traditional Chinese medicine. Many of the techniques used are similar, however, "wet" cupping involves making small incisions in the skin to let blood and interstitial fluids drain. Dry cupping does not require a skin incision whereas wet cupping does. It is believed to assist removing impurities like toxins, and impure blood and tissue fluids. This cupping technique should exclusively be performed by expert practitioners. The procedure can be risky without proper training and without taking the appropriate sanitary precautions as described throughout Chapter 5. Glass cups are normally used for this technique. The equipment needs to be properly cleaned and glass best allows for this.

Wet cupping is sometimes referred to as *Hijama* and has been used for years to improve the natural immune system and cure a variety of disorders. Islamic cultures have long used the practice for healing as the Islamic prophet, Muhammad, recommended the therapy throughout his teachings and writings.

Wet cupping starts in a similar fashion as dry cupping. The area to be treated should be appropriately cleaned and then dried. Many practitioners then start with a dry run to enhance blood flow. This means no incision is made in the skin at first and a patient undergoes dry cupping for the first 5 to 10 minutes of a session. The cups are then removed, and the area is cleaned and wiped down again. A practitioner will then carefully pierce the epidermis a few times with a scalpel. The cups are placed over the small incisions, and the vacuum effect allows for impurities to escape the body.

The cups are left stationary for around 10 minutes and then carefully removed, along with all the blood and toxins. This technique is believed to be highly effective in recovery from injuries or pains, inflammation, and the removal of impurities.

Needle Cupping

Needle cupping is another cupping technique that requires minimal punctures to skin. Unlike wet cupping, however, it will not cause any bloodletting. Needle cupping is the combination of acupuncture and cupping therapy in a single practice. The benefits of combining both treatments include bringing *Qi* along with improved blood flow to different acupuncture points. This helps combat infections like the flu and assists circulation to areas that are in pain. This procedure should not be practiced by novices as it also requires proper cupping therapy training along with acupuncture training. Needle cupping typically requires large glass cups. They need to be large enough to not interfere with the acupuncture needles.

Just as with all cupping techniques, needle cupping requires the area to be treated to be properly cleaned first. After the area is cleaned and dried, a practitioner will insert an acupuncture needle into an appropriate point. A cup is then placed directly on top of the needle with a weak to medium level of suction. Suction should not be overly strong as it will interfere with the acupuncture needle. Strong suction risks removing the needle or forcing it deeper inside a patient. Just as with dry cupping, the cups can be left stationary on a patient for around 10 to 30 minutes.

The practice is said to help break down trigger points, tight muscle, along with sources of pain for patients. An expert practitioner will use the technique to deactivate any trigger point of a patient's pain and help restore normal length and function to poorly circulating muscle.

Flash Cupping

This unique form of the therapy requires a lot of activity from the practitioner. Flash cupping is named appropriately as the process is quick. A practitioner will attach and remove a cup almost immediately and repeat this to a specific area for around 5 minutes.

This technique is believed to be great for weaker patients who need a boost to their energy and Qi. Although the cups only suction skin for seconds at a time, the process still brings nutrients to muscles and so assists healing. Flash cupping will not cause a lot of bruise marks to show as the cups are attached and removed quickly.

After the treatment area on a patient is properly cleaned a practitioner will simply begin the therapy by quickly placing the cups on and off a patient. Depending on the suction method used, the cups may get hot. In this case it is important to have more cups on hand so the patient does not burn. Alternate between cups and repeat the process for up to 5 minutes in a specific area.

As mentioned before, this is a great treatment option for weaker patients. It provides the perfect energy boost and promotes the removal of infections like colds.

Moving Cupping

Moving cupping is another technique that requires a lot of activity from a practitioner. The method is mostly used on larger, flat surfaced parts of the body like the back and legs. It is best to not perform this procedure over bony areas like the knees and elbows as it can be uncomfortable to the patient. This technique is very similar to a massage.

A practitioner will clean the area to be worked on and then apply a therapeutic massage oil. Next, a cup is applied to the skin with a medium to strong suction. The cup is then slid along muscles, and acupuncture points. The suction cannot be too light as movement may cause the cup to pop off. On the other hand suction cannot be too strong as it may prevent the cup from moving. Practitioners will generally use either glass or silicone cups for this technique. These materials can slide comfortably over skin without harming or hurting a patient.

The technique generally lasts around 5 minutes, which allows appropriate blood flow and the lymphatic system to unblock. It is excellent for muscle aches and pain. Lactic acid builds up in muscle which causes pain and moving cupping allows the deep tissues to relax and excrete this chemical.

Fascia holds together the entire body. When healthy it is flexible, glides, and is supple. It allows us to move pain free. For a lot of us this isn't the case and moving cupping helps promote fascia health. The cupping technique releases tension and eases any pain.

Herbal Cupping

Herbal cupping is a technique that has been practiced for years in traditional Chinese medicine. Traditional bamboo cups are boiled in a specific herbal blend. The kinds of herbs used are dependent on what needs to be treated. For kidney health, liver health, and different infections, specified herbs are used.

A practitioner will soak bamboo cups in a herbal blend which allows the bamboo to absorb the different healing properties. After the bamboo cups have absorbed all the proper ingredients, the normal "dry" cupping process takes place. A specific area is treated, and the power of cupping is combined with herbal healing. Cups will remain stationary on a patient for 15 to 30 minutes depending on suction strength.

This technique only applies to practitioners who have an extensive knowledge in herbal health along with cupping using bamboo cups. Bamboo cups are the most challenging cups to use for the therapy. They can have sharp entry points which can damage a patient's skin if suction strength is too strong. The combination of cupping therapy and herbal healing can prove to have many health benefits for patients. It is believed to help chronic pains along with illnesses.

Water Cupping

Most individuals learning about cupping therapy often confuse water cupping with "wet" cupping. The two techniques are very different. Water cupping requires no skin incisions, it simply consists of adding water to cups before they are applied to a patient's skin.

An experienced practitioner will add water to cups until they are around 1/3rd full. Cups are then applied to a patient in a quick matter so that no water is spilled during the process. The cups remain stationary on the patient for 15 to 30 minutes depending on suction strength. Water cupping can be performed at any of the suction strengths discussed earlier in the chapter.

Depending on what needs to be treated or what benefits a patient is looking for, the water used during the technique can either be warm or cool. The process assists the body in either warming up or cooling down. Patients dealing with a cold or with muscle pains that need heating will gain benefits from warm water. Those with any inflammations, or high fevers will benefit from cool water.

Water cupping is believed to help hydrate the body. Patients dealing with hydration issues such as dry throat and skin may see benefits from water cupping.

Glass cups are usually used for this technique, however, plastic or silicone cups can also be used. It is important that the cups are appropriately sealed. Water cupping requires much training as it is important not to spill water inside of a cup over a patient.

Observing the variety of techniques involved with cupping therapy demonstrate how widespread the practice is. Cupping evolved from a variety of beliefs and cultures. The techniques mentioned above all differ slightly, as that is how the wisdom of the practice was passed on. It is good to note that the principles behind the therapy remain the same. Different techniques are great to help different ailments.

... Short Interruption

Hey, are you enjoying the book? I'd love to hear your thoughts!

Many readers do not know how hard reviews are to come by, and how much they help an independent author and publisher.

Cupping Therapy

I would be incredibly thankful if you could take just 30 seconds to write a brief review, even if it's just a few sentences!

>Click here to leave a review<

For those who own a physical copy of the book, I would be equally grateful if you did the same by visiting the books product page on Amazon.

Thank you very much for taking the time to share your thoughts!

Chapter 8
PLACEMENTS FOR TREATMENTS - LOCATION PAINS
PLACEMENTS FROM THE NECK, UPPER BACK & CHEST DOWN TO FEET.

Decompressive Therapy

Clinicians treat pain and discomfort through both compressive and decompressive techniques. Cupping is one of the few therapies that takes advantage of decompressive healing techniques. It provides a lifting effect on the skin rather than a compressive force that is experienced in traditional massage therapies. This helps with healing, decreases pain and promotes interstitial flow. The stagnation process of blood flow is reduced and recovery takes place at a faster rate.

Throughout the following chapters we will view a variety of ailments that cupping may help alleviate.

They are organized by specific location pains, illnesses & issues, and lastly beauty treatments.

Location Pains

The following section describes some treatment options for a variety of location-based issues. Cupping therapy may help recovery from pain throughout the entire body. Consider the following chapter for any issues that are location based.

Cupping Therapy

General Neck & Shoulder Pain

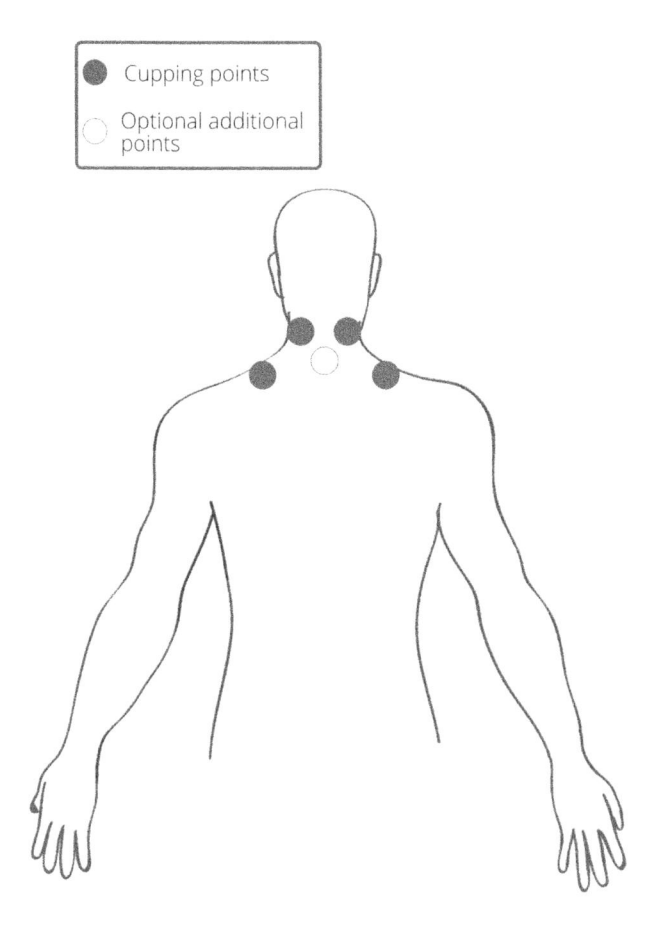

- Cupping points
- Optional additional points

General Neck & Shoulder Pain

There are a variety of classifications when it comes to neck and shoulder pain. Some experience pains only throughout the neck, some only within the shoulders, and for many simultaneous pain is common. This is because the area contains many connective ligaments, nerves, veins, muscles, and other supporting structures that all rely on one another to function smoothly. It is common for an injury effecting one area to have continuous side effects in a variety of other places.

Poor posture along with injury are the biggest culprits when it comes to neck and shoulder pain. Although therapies like cupping can help relief pain, the effects will be temporary if the cause of the pain is from poor posture. It is recommended to visit a clinic that not only offers cupping therapy, however, also works with a patient on improving their posture.

Neck and shoulder pain is often linked to injury of the soft tissue. The injury may come from trauma, muscle strain, poor posture, accidents, or a variety of abnormalities in the bone or joints. An individual is left with discomfort throughout the upper back, which can lead to more symptoms like headaches, stiffness, and constant tiredness.

Cupping may help offer some relief as tension is released and increased blood flow assists the healing process:

- Place 2 cups on the upper part of the neck, at the base of the skull, as shown on the diagram.

- Place 2 more cups on the upper part of the shoulder, close to where the neck begins.

- Optionally place an additional cup just below the base of the neck. This cup may be placed slightly higher up the neck or lower down the spine depending on if a patient's pain is more in the neck area or shoulder area.

- Weak to strong suction may be used. Weak to medium suction for mild pains, and strong suction for acute pain. Leave the cups for stagnant for 10 to 20 minutes. Monitor skin carefully for any adverse side-effects.

- ***Moving cupping** may be used to help treat neck and shoulder pain. Apply only the "optional additional point" cup demonstrated in the diagram and slide the cup up and down the neck, and sideways along the shoulders.

Rotator Cuff

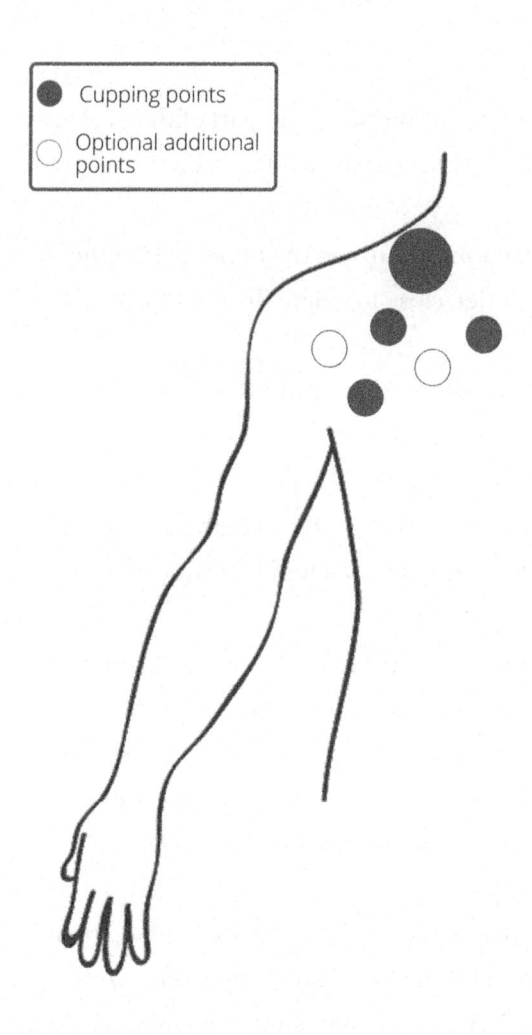

- ● Cupping points
- ○ Optional additional points

Rotator Cuff

The rotator cuff is formed by a group of muscles and tendons whose job it is to keep the arm bone firmly within the socket of the shoulder. This is a vital function that needs to stay healthy as it is required for several daily functions. It is responsible for assisting us with a lot of simple tasks, like combing your hair, or grabbing something off a high shelf.

Injuries or pains to the rotator cuff occur most often in individuals who repeatedly perform overhead motions. The injury is common in baseball, tennis, or swimming, but outside of sports it can also be a frequent ailment.

Injury risks increase as an individual ages and the area experiences greater wear and tear. It can happen suddenly while lifting something heavy, or by falling on your arm. Cupping and getting enough rest may help heal injury to the rotator cuff. Cupping therapy will assist clearing up many of the blockages that may have occurred and increase mobility.

- Place a larger cup at the top of the shoulder as shown on the diagram.

- Next place 3 same sized smaller cups below the

shoulder as shown on the diagram. This helps target the traps, rhomboids, lats teres m, lower rhomboids, and infraspinatus.

- Optionally place 2 additional cups as shown in the diagram for more acute pain.

Frozen Shoulder

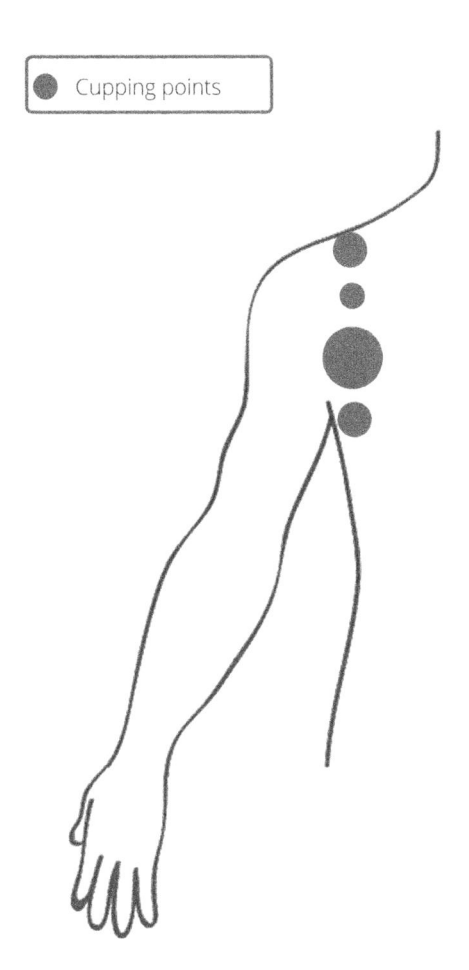

- Cupping points

Frozen Shoulder

Frozen shoulder (*adhesive capsulitis*) is an ailment that limits an individuals range of motion. The condition is characterized by pain and stiffness in the shoulder area. The main cause for frozen shoulder is when the connective tissue that make up the shoulder joint thicken and tighten. This restricts movement and creates a lot of discomfort.

Symptoms and discomfort begin gradually, and slowly continue to get worse. Problems can persist for over 2 years. Unfortunately, it is not clear what causes frozen shoulder.

Cupping may help offer some relief as it potentially increases range of motion and releases the buildup in the area:

- First place a large cup on the deltoid as demonstrated in the diagram.

- Then place a medium size cup just below the first cup on the latissimus dorsi.

- Place another medium size cup at the top of the shoulder straight above the large cup as demonstrated in the diagram.

- Place a last small cup between the top medium cup and the large cup.

- Weak to strong suction may be used. Weak to medium suction for mild pains, and strong suction for acute pain.

MICHAEL L. ZHANG

Shoulder

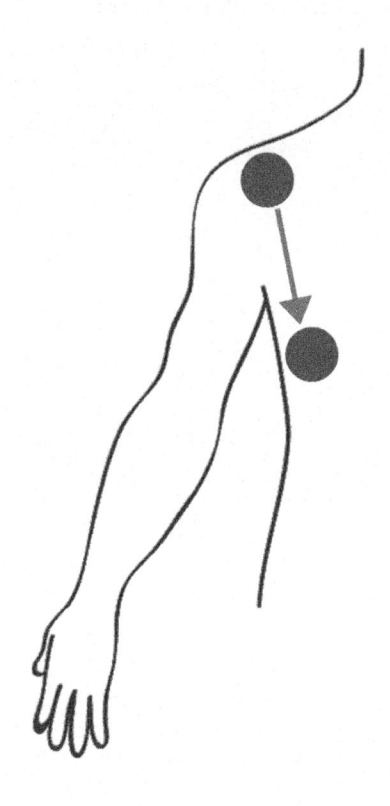

● Cupping points

Shoulder

The shoulder is a complex collection of tendons and muscles that combine with several joints to allow a wide range of motion in the arm. It effects everything from grabbing and lifting things to the simple task of brushing your teeth. Any pain in the shoulder area can make those ordinary things feel like monumental tasks.

Problems in the shoulder are usually caused by impingements of soft tissue in the area and instability. The results are pain, which can be temporary or consistent. There are several ways cupping may help treat general shoulder pain:

- A general treatment option includes static dry cupping. Place a first cup at the top of the shoulder as demonstrated in the diagram.

- Place a second cup on the latissimus dorsi as shown in the diagram.

- Weak to strong suction may be used. Weak to medium suction for mild pains, and strong suction for acute pain.

Moving cupping may also be used to help treat general shoulder pain.

- Place a cup at the top of the shoulder blade.

- Move the cup down and up the shoulder blade area and across the center towards the spine.

- Continue treatment for around 15 minutes.

An active movement technique is also used for treatment. It allows for a more dynamic approach to fascia release, and it allows for greater mobility.

- Place a cup towards upper part of the shoulder as demonstrated in the diagram.

- Ask the patient to move the shoulder into shoulder flexion.

- *Note:* the movement shouldn't be painful. The patient should move up to the point just before pain. Assist the patient into this movement if necessary and repeat the process carefully. Make sure not to push the patient past their limit.

Cupping Therapy

Upper Back

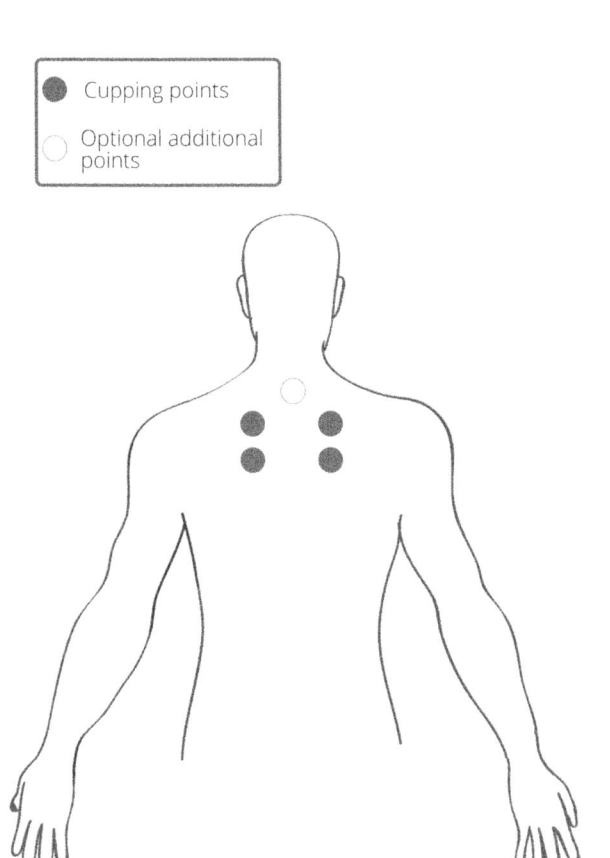

- Cupping points
- Optional additional points

Upper Back

Upper back pain is a common issue for many today. It is often caused by poor posture, injury, or muscle overuse. Issues along the neck and spine can cause a lot of discomfort throughout the rest of the body. The muscles along this area work together and effect many other ligaments and areas. Pain felt in the arms or legs may actually lead back to stress or injury in the neck or spine.

It should be noted that just as we can condition muscles to grow stronger, the opposite is also true. It is possible to decondition our muscles from functioning in the correct manner. This weakens them and causes painful imbalances. Poor posture and remaining seated in unhealthy positions for too long are some of the leading reasons for muscle deconditioning. The result is often discomfort throughout the entire back or upper back.

Cupping may help offer some pain relief and can release a lot of the tension built up in the area:

- Place 4 cups along each side of the spine as demonstrated in the diagram.

Cupping Therapy

- The cups are commonly placed about 1 to 2 inches away from the spine.

- For upper back pain, the cups may be placed higher or lower along the spine depending on where the pain is located.

- Weak to strong suction may be used. Weak to medium suction for mild pains, and strong suction for acute pain.

- Leave the cups stagnant for 10 to 20 minutes.

- An addition cup may be placed just below the neck. This point is usually targeted for stress-related issues and tensions.

Chest

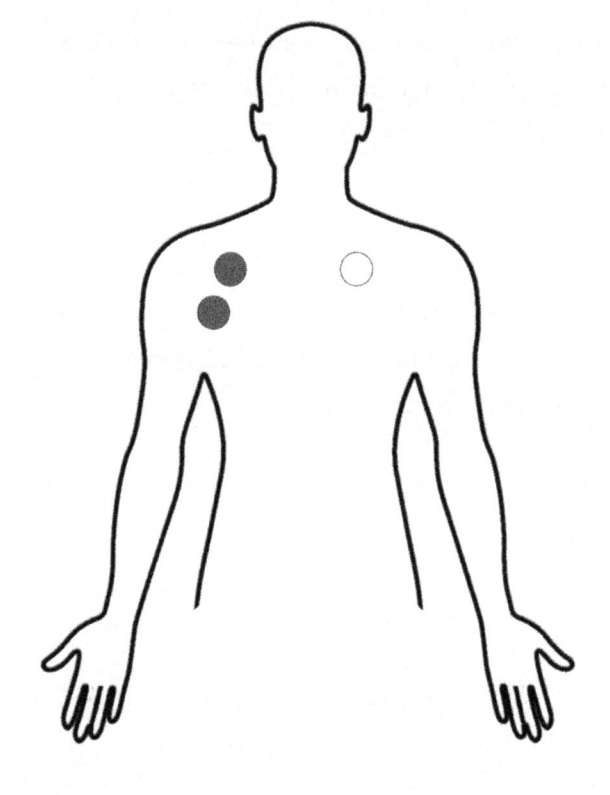

- ● Cupping points
- ○ Optional additional points

Chest

Many worry and relate chest pain with heart issues. Chest pain is certainly something a specialist should look at, however, it involves many possible causes besides the heart. Causes of the pain can be traced back to a variety of problems in the lungs, nerves, ribs, or muscles. These issues may be serious or minor. It is important to have a specialist diagnose the issue and properly identify the source of the pain.

Cupping therapy may help chest pain due to injury or accidents. Poor posture while lifting something heavy can damage soft tissue in the chest area. Lifting the fascia with decompressive therapy can offer a patient some relief.

- Place a cup just below the collarbone on the inside of the shoulder as shown in the diagram.

- Place a second cup just below the first cup, just slightly closer to the armpit.

- Weak to strong suction may be used. Weak to medium suction for mild pains, and strong suction for acute pain.

- Leave the cups stagnant for 10 to 20 minutes.

- An additional cup may be placed below the collarbone in level with a patient's nipples. (As demonstrated in the diagram as "optional additional point")

Moving cupping may be used to help relieve chest pain:

- Place a cup at the "optional additional point" area as demonstrated in the diagram.

- Apply the appropriate suction and slide the cup across the chest and affected areas. Apply treatment for approximately 15 minutes.

Cupping Therapy

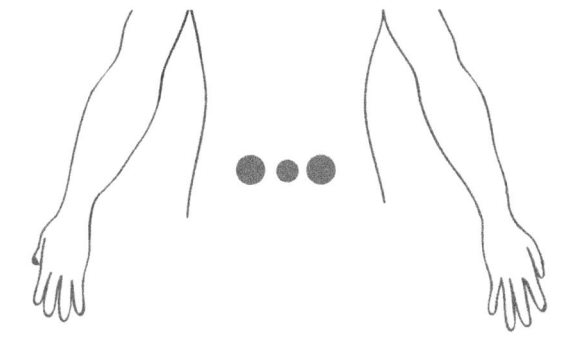

Lower Back

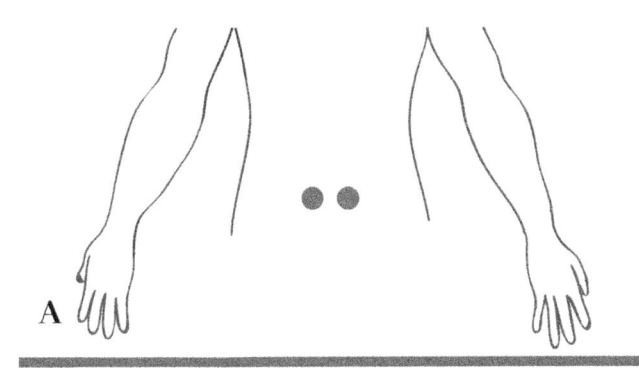

- Cupping points

A

B

Lower Back

Lower back pain is an issue for many. At one point or another, almost everyone deals with issues in this area of the body. The lower area of the spine is a complex structure of interconnecting nerves, joints, ligaments, bones, and muscles all working together as one. It provides everything from flexibility and strength to support. The structure is however susceptible to a variety of injuries and pain. It is in fact the most common cause for missed workdays in the United States of America.

The lower back supports all the weight of the upper body and provides mobility for everyday motions and tasks. The area also supports several functions of the lower body, however. Flexing and rotating the hips are supported by the lower back and this is required for everything from walking to sitting. Next, the nerves in the lower back supply power and sensation to the muscles in the feet and legs.

Pain in the area is typically caused by soft-tissue injuries and mechanical issues. The most common injury is a torn or pulled muscle and/or ligament which causes lower back pain. Cupping can offer some pain relief and be a helpful treatment option. Some practitioners opt to treat lower back pain with flash cupping.

Cupping Therapy

The heat energy created with this technique may speed up the healing process.

There are generally 2 treatment options used, both options are demonstrated in the diagram as A/B.

A

- Place 2 cups on the affected area about 1 inch on the side of the spine as shown in the diagram.

- Weak to strong suction may be used. Weak to medium suction for mild pains, and strong suction for acute pain.

- Leave the cups stagnant for 10 to 20 minutes.

- *Note: Both cups may also be used for moving cupping. Slide both cups up and down the lower back to relieve pain.

B

- Place 2 cups on the lower back about 2.5 inches on the side of the spine as shown in the diagram.

- Place an additional smaller cup directly in between the already placed cups.

- Weak to strong suction may be used. Weak to medium suction for mild pains, and strong suction for acute pain. ***Note:** Patient's with intervertebral discs issues (slipped, herniated) should avoid strong suction and only complete treatment with a specialist.

- Leave the cups stagnant for 10 to 20 minutes.

Cupping Therapy

Full Back

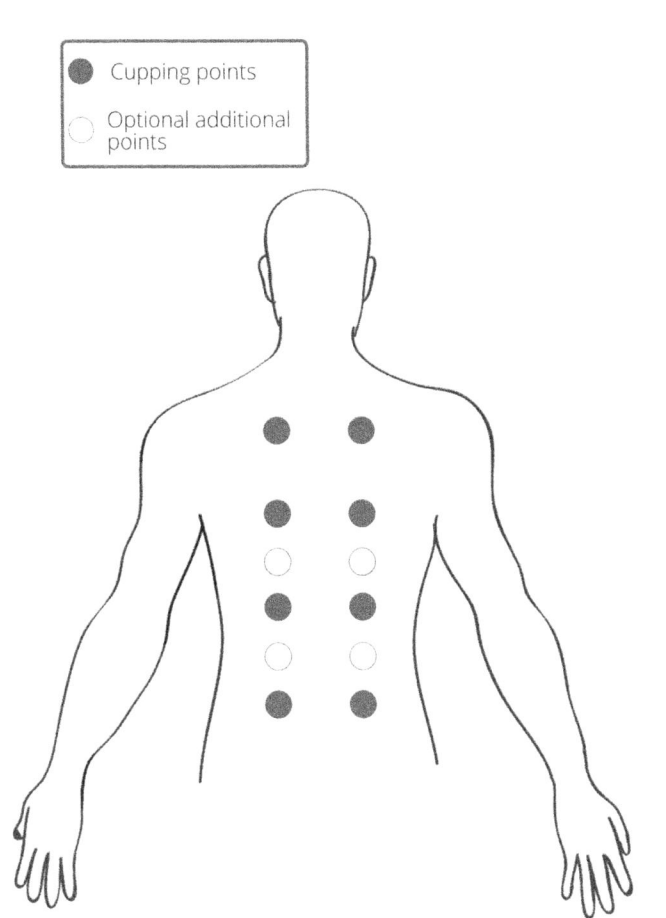

- Cupping points
- Optional additional points

Full Back

The back is an intricate structure of tendons, disks, ligaments, muscles, and bones that work together to support the body and allows movement and flexibility. With that, it is important to keep it in optimal health. It assists the body with so much, and any issues can cause a lot of discomfort.

It is often difficult to determine exactly what causes back pain. Doctors refer to these cases as non-specific back pain. It may come from poor posture, injury, or sprains, but it often happens for no apparent reason. Back pain can lead to additional symptoms such as drowsiness and tingling sensation in various parts of the body.

Cupping on the back may help deal with a variety of pains. Not only does the therapy help with pain relief, it also offers comfort from stress-related back tension. The practice decompresses an area that is almost under constant pressure to support the body.

- Place cups along both sides of the spine (about 2 inches away from the spine) down the full length of a patient's back.

- Weak to strong suction may be used. Weak to

medium suction for mild pains, and
strong suction for acute pain.

- Leave the cups stagnant for 10 to 30 minutes.

- Alternatively, moving cupping may be used. Place 2 cups along each side of the spine and slide the cups up and down a patient's back.

MICHAEL L. ZHANG

Elbow & Forearm

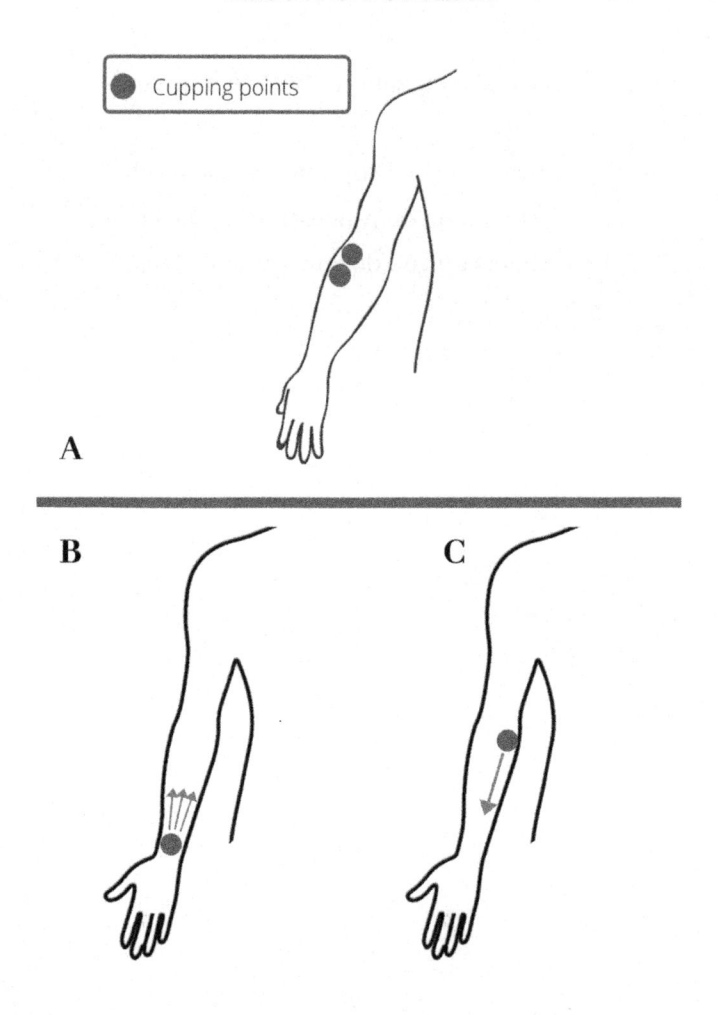

● Cupping points

A

B

C

Elbow & Forearm

The lower section of arms has several smaller bones and ligaments. The area contains a lot of cartilage, ligaments, tendons, nerves, and blood vessels, and if anything happens to these parts, it causes pain. Even with so many variables, the area is quite durable. The joints in the lower section of the arm are much less prone to wear-and-tear damage than many other parts of the body.

Pain in the area is often caused one time injuries. A fall, taking a hit, or lifting something too heavy may cause a sprain or injury. Placing too much stress on the area can lead to damage. Another potential cause for pain may be overuse. In a variety of sports, jobs, and hobbies there is a requirement for repetitive arm, elbow, wrist, or hand movements.

Cupping this area can be a helpful treatment option.

A (treats elbow pain)

- Place a cup just below the point of a patient's elbow (bursa olecranon) as shown in the diagram.

- Place an additional cup just below the previously placed cup.

- Weak to strong suction may be used. Weak to medium suction for mild pains, and strong suction for acute pain.

- Leave the cups stagnant for 5-15 minutes.

B (treats wrist and forearm pain)

- Place a cup on the bottom of a patient's wrist.

- Use moving cupping and slide the cup up and down in 3 directions as shown in the diagram.

- Treat the area for 10 to 15 minutes.

- ***Note:** Use weak to medium cupping for this treatment as strong suction may be uncomfortable at this location.

C (treats elbow and forearm pain)

- Place a cup just below the medial epicondyle on the inside of a patient's arm as shown in the diagram.

- Use moving cupping and slide the cup down and up along the inside of the arm.

- Weak to strong suction may be used. Weak to medium suction for mild pains, and strong suction for acute pain.

- Treat the area for 10 to 15 minutes.

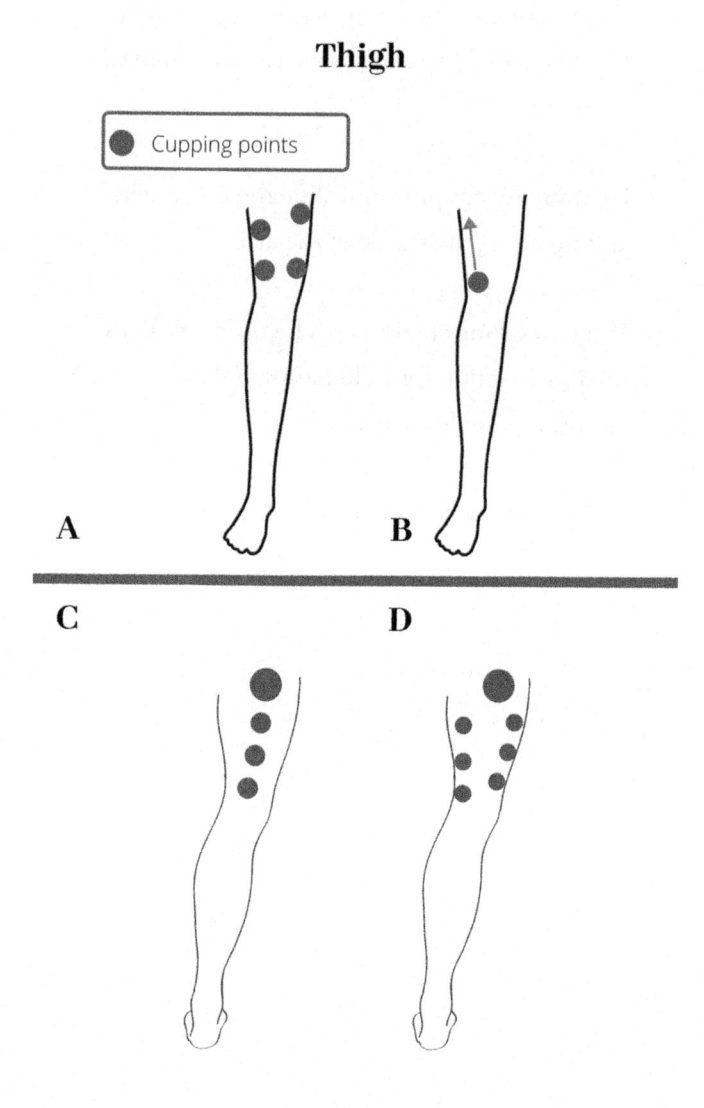

Thigh

- Cupping points

A **B**

C **D**

Thigh

This area of the body has a large number of muscle groups. It is common for thigh pain to derive from (sports) injuries, a variety of conditions, and nerve problems. The pain can range from a mild ache or sharp shooting sensation to chronic pain that can be described as a burning sensation or numbness. The thigh area consists of the hamstrings, quadriceps, and iliotibial (IT band). They allow us to stand, run, climb, and everything in between.

Athletes often strain and/or sprain a muscle, tendon, or ligament in the thigh area. A strain happens when a tendon or muscle is overly stretched or tears. A sprain happens when a ligament is overly stretched or tears. Overuse and under-use are both reasons for these types of injuries to happen. Not warming up before exercise and working out too long or too hard. On the other end of the spectrum is simply not getting enough exercise and spending too much time sitting.

Cupping is a great solution for thigh pain. It may help with injury recovery but also assists with any aches or pains in the area.

. . .

A (treats quadriceps pain)

- Place 2 cups on each side of the quadriceps. 2 along the inside and 2 along the outside as shown in the diagram. The 2 cups on the inner thigh may be positioned slightly higher.

- Weak to strong suction may be used. Weak to medium suction for mild pains, and strong suction for acute pain.

- Treat the area for 10 to 20 minutes.

B (treats the IT band and general thigh area)

- Place a cup slightly above the knee area either on the inner thigh or outer thigh as shown in the diagram.

- Apply weak to strong suction. Weak to medium suction for mild pains, and strong suction for acute pain.

- Slide the cup up and down the IT band or problem ear on the thigh.

- Treat the area for 10 to 20 minutes.

C (treats hamstring pain)

- Place a large cup at the highest end of the hamstring (just on or right below the glutes) as shown in the diagram.

- Place 3 cups directly below the previously placed cup following the sciatic nerves.

- Weak to strong suction may be used. Weak to medium suction for mild pains, and strong suction for acute pain.

- Treat the area for 10 to 20 minutes.

D (treats hamstring pain)

- Place a large cup at the highest end of the hamstring (just on or right below the glutes) as shown in the diagram.

- Place 3 cups along each side of the hamstrings.

3 along the inside and 3 along the outside as shown in the diagram. The 3 cups running along the inner thigh may be positioned slightly higher.

- Weak to strong suction may be used. Weak to medium suction for mild pains, and strong suction for acute pain.

- Treat the area for 10 to 20 minutes.

Cupping Therapy

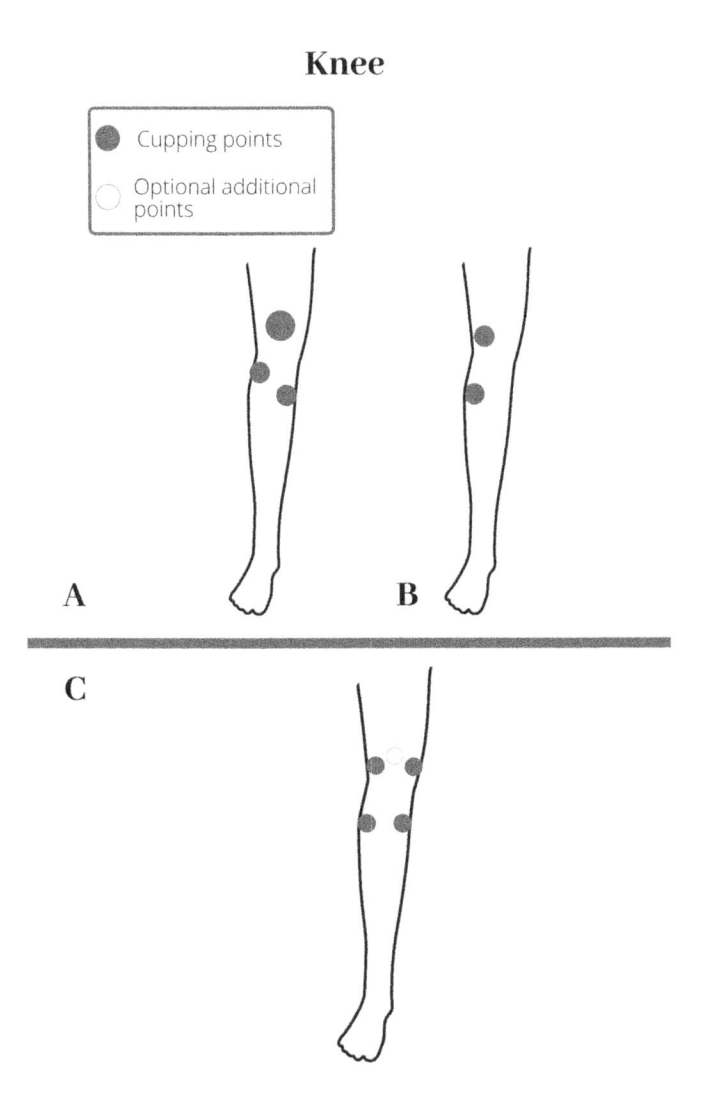

Knee

- Cupping points
- Optional additional points

A

B

C

95

Knee

The knee is the largest supporting joint in the body. The area attaches the thigh with the leg and consists of two joints, the tibiofemoral and the patellofemoral. It allows both flexion and extension along with slight internal and external rotation.

Due to the complexity of the joint, it is susceptible to a few injuries and ailments. Knee pain is common and can affect individuals of all ages. Sports injuries such as ruptured ligaments or torn cartilage are a regular occurrence in the area. These injuries often require surgery to help repair any tears. The road to recovery is usually a long one, as a patient will experience a lot of pain and swelling. This is where cupping may help speed up the healing process. Cupping can be used to reduce inflammation and pain, break down scar tissue, and bring nutrients to the injured area.

A (treats general knee pain)

- Place a large cup on the top of the knee as shown in the diagram.

- Place a smaller cup towards the end of the IT band as shown in the diagram.

- Place a last cup on the inside of the knee or the medial collateral ligament as shown in the diagram.

- Weak to strong suction may be used. Weak to medium suction for mild pains, and strong suction for acute pain.

- Treat the area for 10 to 20 minutes.

B (treats front and lower knee pain)

- Place a cup towards the outside and just above the knee as shown in the diagram. Just above the lateral and superior patellar facets.

- Place a cup directly below the first cup under the knee. Just to the outside of the tibia.

- Weak to strong suction may be used. Weak to medium suction for mild pains, and strong suction for acute pain.

- Treat the area for 10 to 20 minutes.

C (treats general knee pain)

- Place 4 cups surrounding the knee as shown in the diagram.

- An additional cup may be placed above the patella right below the quadriceps.

- Weak to strong suction may be used. Weak to medium suction for mild pains, and strong suction for acute pain.

- Treat the area for 10 to 20 minutes.

Cupping Therapy

Shin Splints

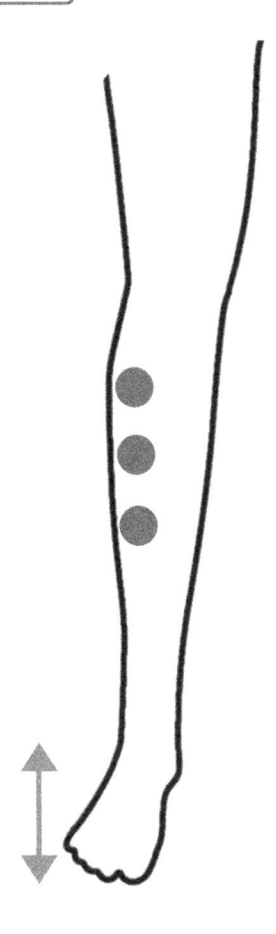

- Cupping points

Shin Splints

Medial tibial stress syndrome... This is what doctors call shin splints. It happens when the shinbone and the connective tissues that attach muscles to the bones in the area are put under too much stress. The result is inflammation and pain.

Some reasons for shin splint are too much exercise, flat feet, and improper lower body support. Furthermore, individuals with weak core muscles, ankles, or hips are at a greater risk for developing shin splints. Treatment options are rest, ice, anti-inflammatories, and cupping may help speed up recovery.

- Place a cup towards the top of the shin on the affected side as shown in the diagram.

- Place 2 more cups directly underneath the previously placed cup.

- Weak to strong suction may be used. Weak to medium suction for mild pains, and strong suction for acute pain.

- Treat the area for 10 to 20 minutes.

- A patient can add movement to further improve rehabilitating the area. Flex the feet in and out of dorsi flexion for 3 to 5 minutes at a time.

Lower Legs

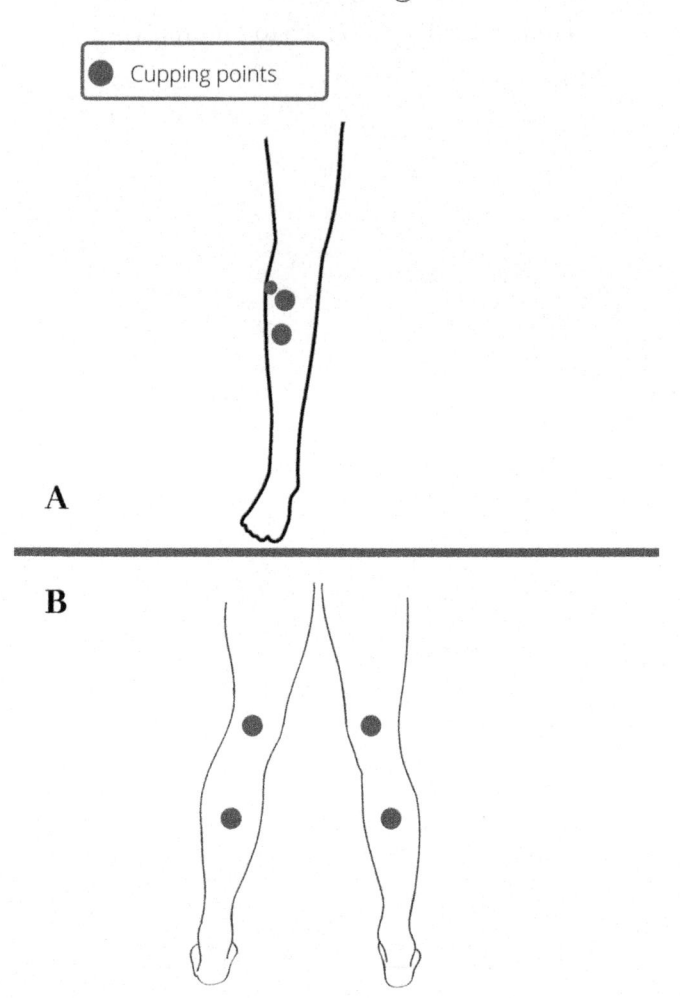

A

B

Lower Legs

Lower leg pain is a common occurrence, however, it can be a challenge finding the specific cause of the issue. The area is responsible for supporting much of our weight and links to many nerves spread throughout the entire body. Common causes for discomfort include muscle strain, injuries, spine problems, and nerve issues.

Visit a healthcare professional for proper diagnosis, however, cupping can be a great way to recover from general soreness and improve the natural healing process.

A (treats frontal lower leg pain)

- Place a cup just below the center of the knee, slightly towards the outside of the tibia.

- Place a second cup directly below the previously placed cup just off of the tibia.

- Place a last smaller cup just next to the first placed cup on the outside of the leg as shown in the diagram.

- Weak to strong suction may be used. Weak to

medium suction for mild pains, and
strong suction for acute pain.

- Treat the area for 10 to 20 minutes.

- Moving cupping may also be used. Place only the first cup and slide the cup down and up the lower leg besides the shin.

B (general treatment of back lower leg area)

- Place a cup on the popliteal fossa, the area opposite of the knee as shown in the diagram.

- Place a second cup directly in the middle of the lower leg between the ankle and knee.

- The popliteal fossa area contains several sensitive nerves so generally weak to medium suction is used on this area. Strong suction can be used however, the area must be monitored carefully.

- Treat the area for 10 to 20 minutes.

- Moving cupping may also be used. Place only the cup on the calf and slide the cup up and down the lower leg.

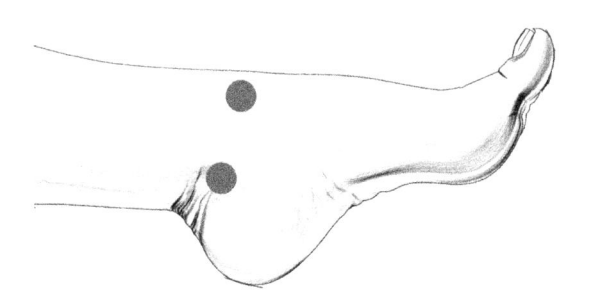

Ankle

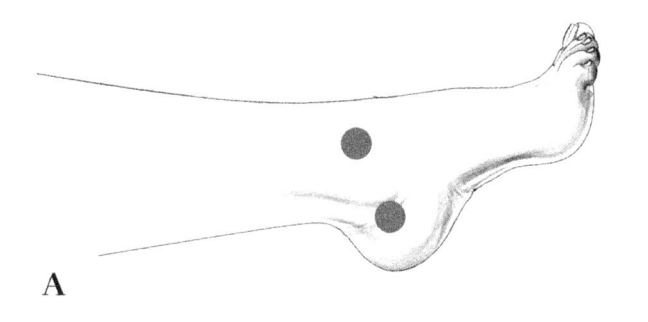

- Cupping points

A

B

Ankle

The ankle is a joint made out of 3 bones, the tibia, fibula, and the talus. The ankle and foot support the weight of the entire body and allows for the up and down, and side-to-side motion of the foot. There are several small bones and ligaments surrounding the ankle, and this means the area risks a variety of small sprains, strains, and tears.

Pain in the area can derive from a variety of sources, however, the main culprits are injury (sprain), instability, and infection. Cupping therapy is a great way to further enhance the natural healing process.

A (treats outer (lateral) ankle pain)

- Place 2 cups along the bottom and upper side of the lateral malleolus (end of the fibula). View diagram for placement.

- Use appropriately sized cups and weak to medium suction.

- Treat the area for 10 to 20 minutes.

B (treats inner (medial) ankle pain)

- Place 2 cups slightly below the medial malleolus (end of the tibia) as shown in the diagram.

- Use appropriately sized cups and weak to medium suction.

- Treat the area for 10 to 20 minutes.

MICHAEL L. ZHANG

Feet

- Cupping points

A

B

108

Feet

The feet support the entire body and allow us to do everything from stand, walk, and jump. They consist of flexible structures of joints, muscles, bones, and soft tissue. These elements all allow for complex movements needed for motion and balance.

With so many factors at play, there are risks for injury. Foot pain can originate from injury, overuse, and inflammation. Cupping the feet can assist the recovery process and relief some tension that is often present in that area. It will improve circulation and help with inflammation and releasing the fascia.

A (static foot treatment option)

- Place a larger cup on the heel of the foot or the calcaneus as shown in the diagram.

- Place a smaller cup along the middle of the foot.

- Place a last cup towards the ball of the foot.

- Use appropriately sized cups and weak to medium suction.

- Treat the area for around 10 minutes.

B (treats general foot pain)

- Place a cup on the ball of the foot, and slide it up and down towards the heel.

- Use medium suction and treat the area for around 10 minutes.

Chapter 9
PLACEMENTS FOR TREATMENTS - ILLNESSES & ISSUES
COMMON ISSUES CUPPING HELPS RESOLVE.

The following section describes some treatment options for a variety of illnesses and issues. Cupping therapy may help recovery from headaches, stomach issues, virus infections, allergies, and much more. Consider the following chapter for illnesses or issues that are not location dependent.

Tension & Headaches

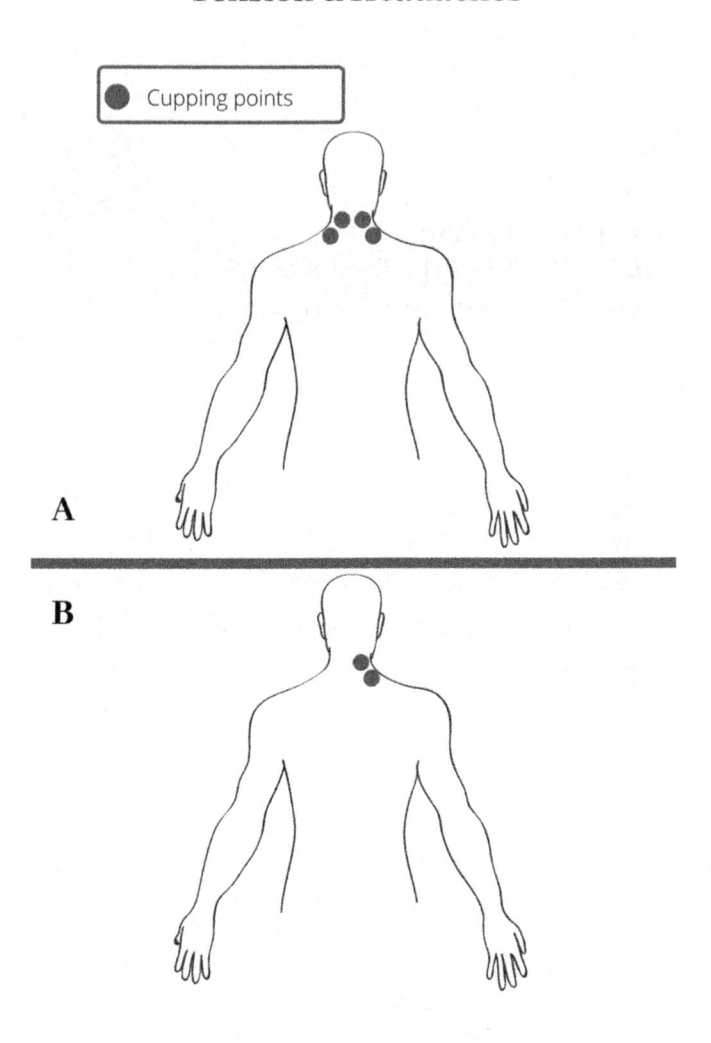

A

B

Tension & Headaches

A tension type headache is very uncomfortable. Life's pressures can put a lot of stress on an individual, and eventually the body will let you know to take things a bit easier. Feelings of mild to intense pain behind the eyes or forehead are common. Furthermore, tension will be present throughout the head, neck, and back.

Cupping may offer some relief, helping a patient relax, and decompress some pressure points around the neck and shoulders.

A (general cupping to help release tension)

- Place 2 cups near the top of the neck below the hairline as shown in the diagram.

- Place 2 cups just below the previously placed points to target the shoulders.

- Weak to strong suction may be used. Weak to medium suction for relaxation, and strong suction for relieving tension.

- Leave the cups stagnant up to around 20 minutes.

B (general cupping to help release tension)

- Target one side at a time by placing 1 cup on the right side by the top of the neck and 1 cup just below it targeting the right shoulder.

- Weak to strong suction may be used. Weak to medium suction for relaxation, and strong suction for relieving tension.

- Leave the cups stagnant up to around 20 minutes.

- While treating one side, a practitioner can gently massage the other side to combine the treatment with massage.

Cupping Therapy

Stomach Issues

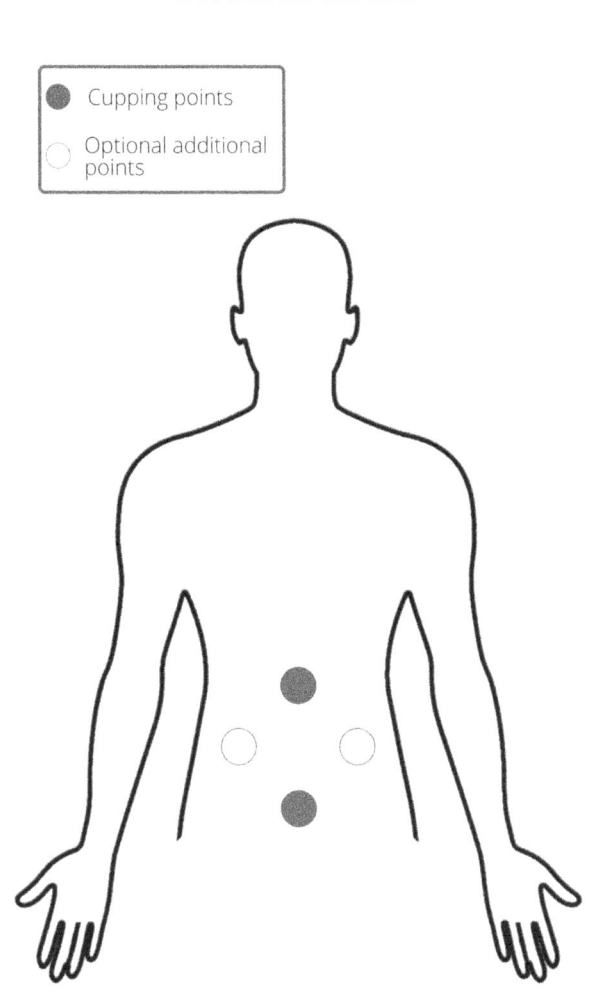

- ● Cupping points
- ○ Optional additional points

Stomach Issues

Stomachaches are a common issue that everyone experiences at one point or another. Most issues are not a serious cause for concern, however the feeling is generally uncomfortable and annoying. If symptoms last abnormally long, and continue to worsen, it is best to consult with a professional to investigate the cause.

Stomach issues are generally related to eating something that does not sit well, inflammations, or disorders. Cupping may help with a variety of stomach issues from bloating to constipation to general discomfort.

***Note:** Pregnant women should avoid cupping in this area.

- Place a cup in the center of the body about 2 inches below the navel.

- Place a cup in the center of the body about 2 inches above the navel.

- Optionally add 2 additional cups, one on each side of the navel as shown in the diagram.

- Weak to medium suction may be used.

- Leave the cups stagnant for up to 15 minutes.

- Moving cupping may also be used. Place a cup about 2 inches above the navel, and slowly slide it in a counterclockwise direction around the navel.

Cold

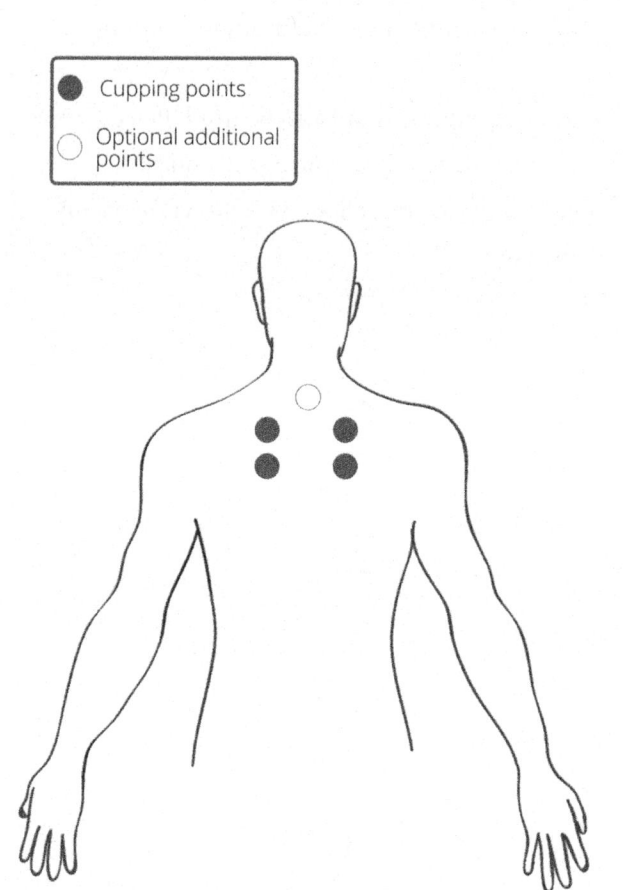

- ● Cupping points
- ○ Optional additional points

Cold

The common cold is a viral infection of the upper respiratory tract (nose and throat). The viruses can be transmitted by direct contact with infected secretions or by virus-infected airborne droplets. This makes the sickness easy to pick up, and it is not abnormal for healthy adults to have up to 3 colds annually.

A cold is ordinarily harmless and recovery usually takes less than 2 weeks. The side effects of a cold may make those days feel much longer, however. A sore throat, coughing, congestion, body aches, headaches, and fever are all common symptoms. Cupping may assist the body in getting rid of a cold. The therapy can flush the system of the virus and help boost the immune system.

- Place 4 cups on the upper back, about 2 inches to either side of the spine as shown in the diagram.

- Place an additional optional cup along the spine just below the neck.

- Medium to strong suction may be used.

- Leave the cups stagnant up to around 15 minutes.

- ***Note:** Some practitioners will use moving cupping on the chest to help combat a cold. Slide a cup along the chest to help relieve congestion from the area.

Cupping Therapy

Allergies

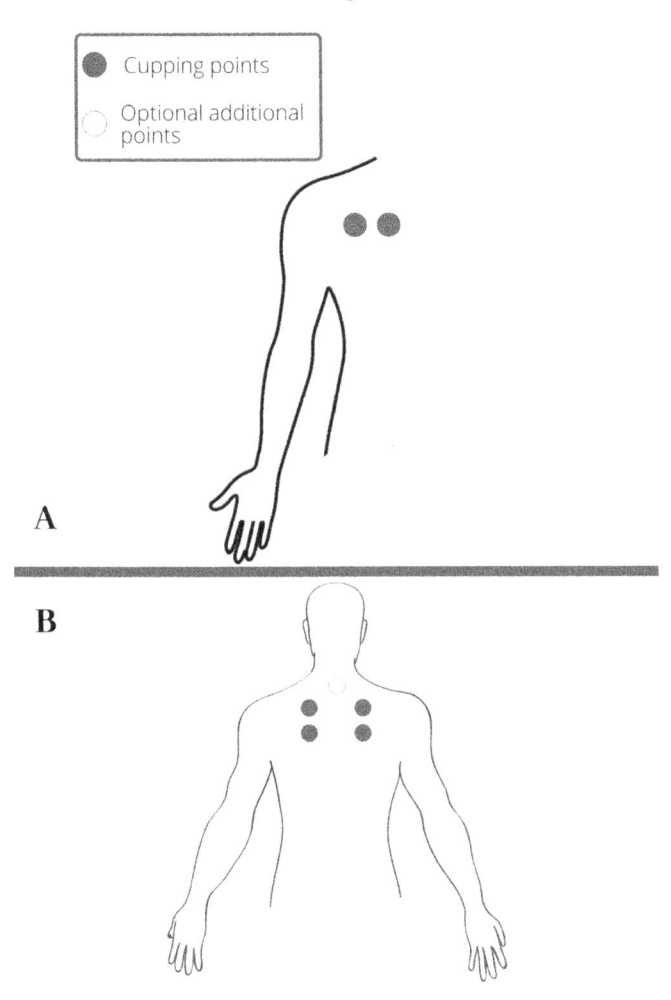

- Cupping points
- Optional additional points

A

B

Allergies

Allergies are a response from our immune system to a foreign substance it considers potentially harmful. Our immune system's job is to keep us healthy, and so it creates different reactions to help fight harmful pathogens. Allergies are not typically harmful, however, it signifies that our body does not react well to these substances. Substances can include different foods, pollen, stings, pets, dust, and many others. When these substances come into touch with the antibodies running through our system, reactions can break out in the form of inflammation on the skin, airways, digestive system, and sinuses.

Unfortunately, most allergies can't be cured, however there are treatments that may help relieve some of the symptoms. Cupping is a great therapy of the immune system that can help flush the system and with recovery from allergy symptoms.

A (assists immune system recovery and chest congestion)

- Place 2 cups next to each other on the chest about 2 inches above the nipples as shown in the diagram.

- Apply weak to medium suction up to around 10 minutes.

- Alternatively, use only 1 cup and apply moving cupping across the chest. Slide the cups in an outward direction.

B (assists immune system recovery, relaxation, air flow, and tension release)

- Place 4 cups on the upper back, about 2 inches to either side of the spine as shown in the diagram.

- Place an additional optional cup along the spine just below the neck.

- Weak to strong suction may be used.

- Leave the cups stagnant up to around 15 minutes.

Air Flow

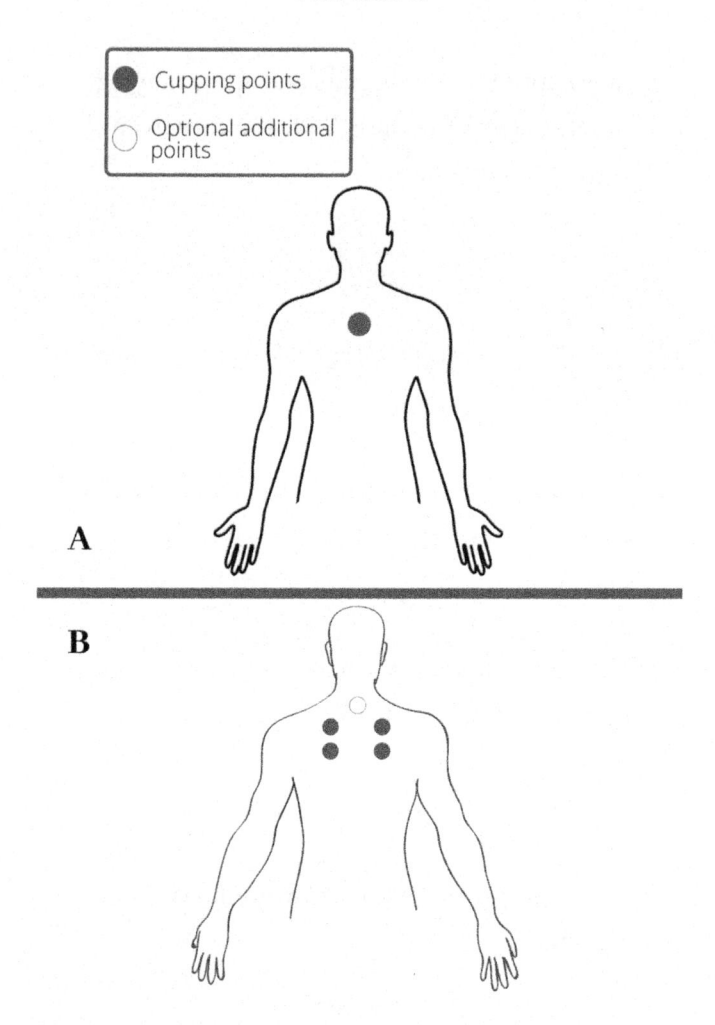

A

B

Air Flow

Breathing is a critical however often ignored activity. Obviously we don't actively think about the task. It would be very dangerous if we constantly had to think about the activity. Actively controlling our breath, however, can be very powerful. It improves physical and mental performance, helps with energy, sleep, stress, illness, and much more.

Air is an amazing force that flushes through the entire body and helps keep us healthy and strong. Cupping may help enhance what the breath does within our bodies naturally. It assists with blood flow and relaxes tension buildup within the body. In traditional Chinese medicine there is believed to be Qi energy running through us. Cupping helps enhance this energy and subsequently improves breathing and airflow.

A (air flow)

- Place one cup at the center of the chest as shown in the diagram.

- Use weak to medium suction.

- Leave the cup stagnant for 5 to 10 minutes.

- Alternatively, use moving cupping up and down the center of the chest.

B (assists immune system recovery, relaxation, air flow, and tension release)

- Place 4 cups on the upper back, about 2 inches to either side of the spine as shown in the diagram.

- Place an additional optional cup along the spine just below the neck.

- Weak to strong suction may be used.

- Leave the cups stagnant up to around 15 minutes.

Cupping Therapy

Stress & Anxiety

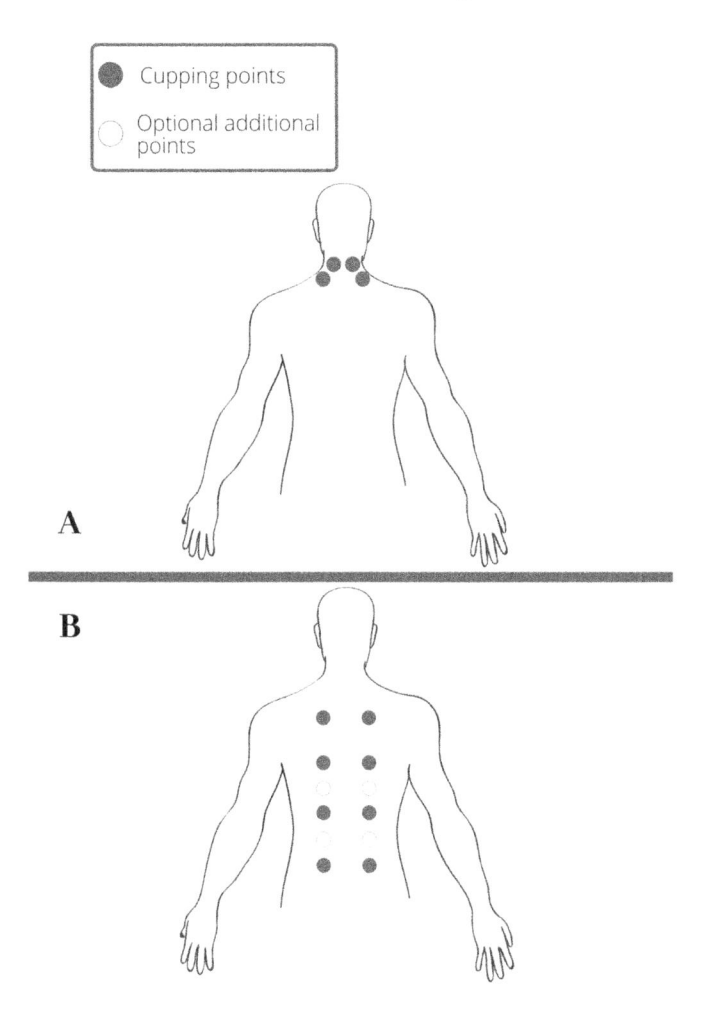

- Cupping points
- Optional additional points

A

B

Stress & Anxiety

Stress and anxiety can be incredibly detrimental to health and wellbeing. Most experience periods of stress and anxiety from time to time. It can show up in various forms as it can be defined as any demand placed on the body or brain. It is easy for this to happen, as today we often deal with multiple competing demands. Anxiety and stress generally show up together. Anxiety is a feeling of worry or fear that may be a reaction of stress.

The feeling of stress and anxiety are actually defense mechanisms. This means they are not always bad, as they can help us escape potentially dangerous situations and challenges. The problem comes when we are under constant pressure. Constant worrying with no release or quiet times can lead to larger issues. The immune system will begin to suffer, and so does our health. Cupping may help ease some of the built up tension and help relieve some stress and anxiety.

A (release tension)

- Place 2 cups near the top of the neck below the hairline as shown in the diagram.

- Place 2 cups just below the previously placed points to target the shoulders.

- Weak to strong suction may be used. Weak to medium suction for relaxation, and strong suction for relieving tension.

- Leave the cups stagnant up to around 20 minutes.

B (general relaxation and improved back health)

- Place cups along both sides of the spine (about 2 inches away from the spine) down the full length of a patient's back.

- Weak to strong suction may be used. Weak to medium suction for mild pains, and strong suction for acute pain.

- Leave the cups stagnant for 10 to 30 minutes.

- Alternatively, moving cupping may be used. Place 2 cups along each side of the spine and slide the cups up and down a patient's back.

Chapter 10
PLACEMENTS FOR TREATMENTS - BEAUTY
SKIN CARE TREATMENTS

The following section describes how cupping therapy can be added to a beauty routine. Cupping has been said to not only promote healing but also cell repair which can aid regeneration. Beauticians have used this to help reduce and remove stretch marks, wrinkles, and other skin ailments. Consider the following chapter for any cupping beauty treatments.

Skin Health

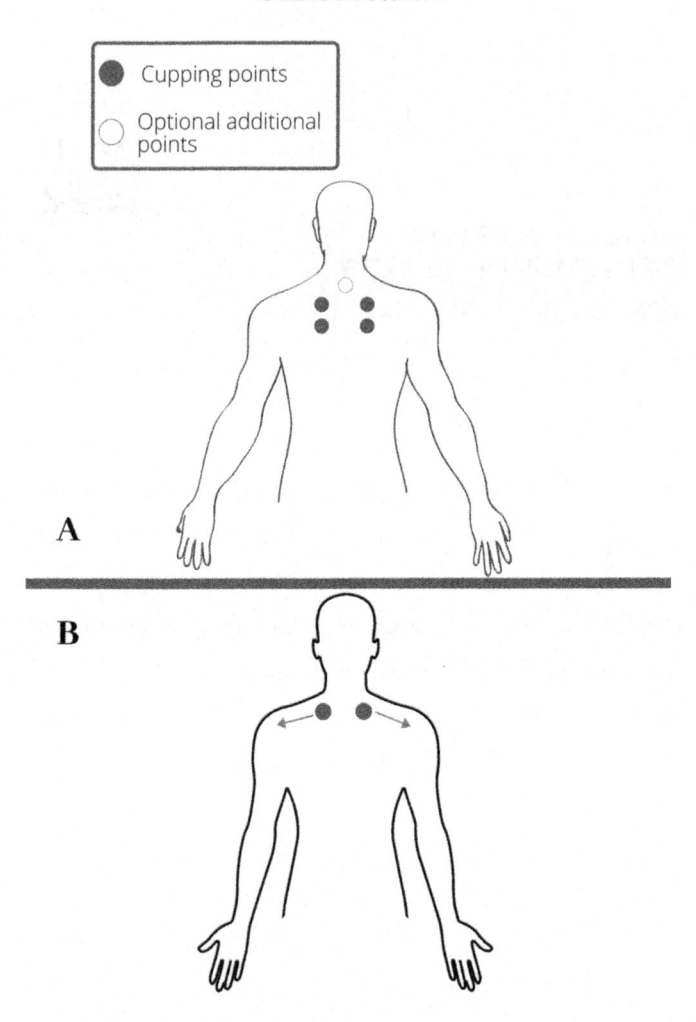

- ● Cupping points
- ○ Optional additional points

A

B

Skin Health

Skin is the first layer of defense against the outside world. The organ (it is the body's largest organ) protects us from viruses, pollution, bacteria, and chemical substances that come across our path daily. Besides protection skin maintains fluid balance, regulates body temperature, acts as a barrier, and recognizes pain sensations to keep us safe. Given all of these vital roles, it is equally important to keep skin healthy.

There are a variety of ways to help skin looking and working at it's best. Properly hydrating, eating a well-balanced diet, reduced stress, proper sleep, and moisturizing are just a view ways of keeping skin supple and healthy. Cupping therapy may help by bringing nutrients to skin cells. The practice can also help smoothen out wrinkles and scarring and helps the body's overall health.

A (general health)

- Place 4 cups on the upper back, about 2 inches to either side of the spine as shown in the diagram.

- Place an additional optional cup along the spine just below the neck.

- Medium to strong suction may be used.

- Leave the cups stagnant up to around 15 minutes.

B (circulation & general health)

- Place 2 cups in line with the end of the neck, below the collarbone as shown in the diagram.

- Use moving cupping and slide the cups outwards towards the shoulders.

- Weak to medium suction may be used.

- Treat the area for up to around 10 minutes.

Cupping Therapy

Wrinkles & Skin Care

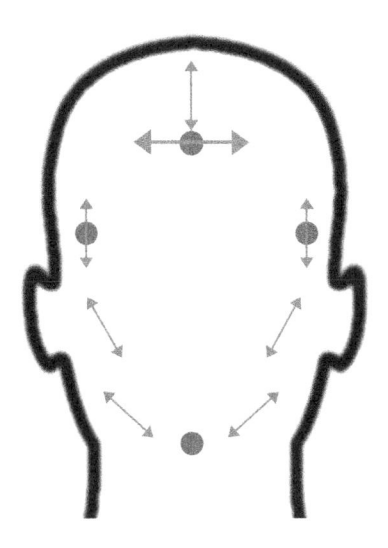

● Cupping points

Wrinkles & Skin Care

Skin tells the stories of our lives. Sunspots, aging, acne scars... they all reflect our age and health, and it's all reflected in our skin. Wrinkles and other marks on the skin are a natural part of the aging process. As we age skin gets less elastic, drier, thinner, and shows signs of maturing.

A good skin care routine can help keep skin looking healthy and vibrant for longer. Cupping can be great to add to that routine as it may help reduce wrinkles, and scars caused by acne. Special cups are required for cupping in the face. They are typically smaller and softer, however, the general techniques used are the same. Facial cupping rarely leaves bruises, but if a cup is left stagnant for too long, there is the risk of a mark being left behind.

Cupping may produce several benefits as it stimulates the cells responsible for collagen production, relaxes muscle tension, strengthens skin, and increases blood circulation in the area. This all can help brighten skin and minimize the appearance of scars, wrinkles, and fine lines.

- Place cups in areas of the face where wrinkles

are present. The diagram shows common areas where fine lines may be present.

- Use moving cupping to slide a cup over areas you want to treat.

- Weak to medium suction may be used.

- Treat specific areas for up to 5 minutes at a time.

Stretch Marks & Cellulite

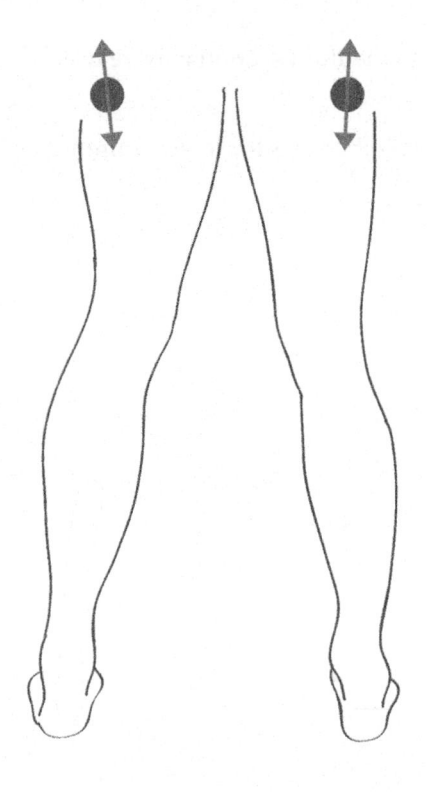

- Cupping points

Stretch Marks & Cellulite

The dimples and marks in skin caused by cellulite, and stretch marks are perfectly normal. Cellulite is actually developed in the layer of fat that exists between skin and muscle. It is not a sign of being unhealthy; it is simply a buildup that pushes against the skin while muscle cords pull downward. This causes an appearance of dimples on the skin's surface. Strech marks appear when the skin tries to adapt to your body. As your body grows or changes, skin is not always able to grow at the same speed. Again, this is not necessarily a sign of being unhealthy.

Cupping may help treat the appearance of cellulite and stretch marks. The practice can help bring nutrients to the area and stimulate collagen production. Furthermore, it brings blood flow to the problem areas and improve lymphatic drainage.

- Place a cup on the area you wish to treat (hips, arms, thighs, etc.).

- Use moving cupping to slide a cup over problem areas.

- Treat a small area for a minimum of 5 minutes at a time.

- Weak to strong suction may be used depending on what area is being treated.

Chapter 11

AFTER THERAPY

NOW WHAT?

Some patients are uneasy about undergoing the therapy. Cupping is not painful, and with a trained practitioner, the practice is safe and relaxing. In most cases a patient is more relaxed when they understand what to expect in a session.

If a patient doesn't suffer from any of the issues discussed in Chapter 4, they are free to experience all the benefits of the practice. The most commonly treated areas are the back, shoulders, neck, and legs. Different locations require different sized cups, along with different amounts of cups.

The Feeling

Depending on the suction and cupping technique, the

feeling of the practice varies slightly. In most cases a patient will feel warmth from the glass on their skin. The suction is described to be comfortable. As time passes, the suction may slowly gain strength. Depending on a patient's condition and what needs to be treated, 1 to over 10 cups may be used.

It is common for a combination of smaller and larger cups to be used at once. Larger fleshier areas will be treated with larger cups, and smaller, more intricate parts of the body with smaller cups. The treatment allows for blood to circulate the area and improve functions of the body. A practitioner will continue to monitor the cups carefully to ensure appropriate suction and to observe discoloration and changes to the skin. A trained practitioner in traditional Chinese medicine can observe the changes in coloration on the skin to determine if there are any stagnations or issues in the area.

Cups are generally not left on the skin for longer than a maximum of 30 minutes. It is dependent on suction strength and what needs to be treated. Removing cups is a painless process and is often followed by small massage, or continued treatment. Some patients describe a light tingling sensation in the treated area, which is normal and healthy.

It is common for some bruising to occur after a session.

Most bruising disappears within a week, but on some patients the discoloration may last longer. Although the bruising has a powerful appearance, the area itself will not be tender or painful. They are simply cupping beauty marks.

Post Session Protocol

After a session at a clinic or at home, it is important to hydrate properly. Cupping therapy helps release toxins and blood flow. A patient can assist the body flush out toxins by drinking plenty of water. Muscle tissue has been lifted and allowed to relax, drinking water will allow those areas to be properly hydrated and supple.

After a session, it is best to simply follow your regular routine. Athletes looking to use the therapy can organize a session around regular routines. It is best to not undergo a procedure for the first time right before a big event. Cupping therapy is often used as a complimentary treatment, so it is great for athletes to use it in this manner. If you are experiencing tightness in an area or compromised movement, it is great to schedule a session to treat the area. Minor improvements that allow for better mobility and an improved workout are felt right away.

For 24 hours after cupping, the following activities should be avoided:

- **Sunbathing:** It is best to avoid direct sunlight on the treated and bruised areas.

- **Sauna & Hot Tub:** Avoid extreme temperature conditions, either hot or cold. Hot showers or baths should also be avoided.

- **Intense Exercise:** Athletes that often undergo the procedure can continue regular activity, however, in most cases it is best to follow regular routines.

- **Heavy, Unhealthy Meals:** Cupping helps release toxins, allow the body to flush the system. Eating heavy and unhealthy meals places many of these toxins right back into the body.

Clearing up the Bruise

Bruising is a natural side effect of cupping therapy. The coloration within bruises show a variety of health conditions of a patient. Cupping allows different toxins to be drawn upwards and these can be visible in the marks on an individuals skin. The body can flush out these toxins quickly after a session and the bruises left behind typically disappear within a week. Depending on a patient's health along with suction strength, the marks left behind may remain longer or shorter.

It is important to distinguish the differences between a bruise resulting from an injury and the marks left behind from cupping therapy. The marks left after cupping are not painful and do not hurt when touched or rubbed. The marks are created by fluids moving towards the surface of skin versus the traditional bruise that is created by a collision which tears blood vessels. Cupping marks are therefore not an actual bruise.

It is possible to speed up the recovery of cupping marks. There are some steps a patient can take that help the body flush out buildup of fluids in an area. Cupping marks can be relieved by following the steps below:

- Rehydrate:

The week following a session, it is crucial to stay hydrated. Water or infused water is best as it helps the body eliminate toxins and replenish.

. . .

- <u>Eat healthy & balanced meals</u>:

An individual's diet has a tremendous impact on all areas of health. Eating well-balanced meals allows the body the heal, flush out toxins, strengthen blood vessels (which further assists blood flow generated by cupping therapy), and creates strong, pliable tissues. Consider adding the following foods to your diet to potentially help clear up bruising more quickly:

- **Citrus Fruits:** Oranges, tangerines, and lemons all have anti-inflammatory properties and contain natural quercetin which promoteshealing.

- **Foods with vitamin K:** This vitamin helps control the binding of calcium on bones along with blood clot. Natural sources are found in broccoli, Brussels sprouts, spinach, kale, soybeans, lettuce, blueberries, and strawberries.

- **Pineapple:** Pineapples contain a mixture of enzymes called bromelain. This helps reduce inflammation and is a great fruit to add to a diet.

- **Lean proteins:** Proteins help re-build muscle

tissue and strengthen capillaries. Not all proteins are optimal. Avoid sources with high amounts of saturated fats and cholesterol often found in fried meats. Great options include lean meat, fish, poultry, tofu, and even vegetables like watercress, spinach, and asparagus.

- Zinc-rich foods: Zinc assists the body heal muscle tissue. Zinc can be found in spinach, legumes, pumpkin seeds, crab, and lobster.

- <u>Massage & Ointments:</u>

Massaging the marks will encourage the breakdown of fluid buildup in the area and allow the marks to disappear faster. Start massaging the middle of the mark in a circular motion and slowly work outwards. An additional step that may be helpful is to combine the massage with either pure aloe vera gel or pure pineapple juice. Aloe vera and pineapple reduce inflammation and may help heal bruising. It is best to use pure ingredients with no additives.

THANK YOU!

Thank you very much for supporting my work. I am incredibly grateful that you finished reading the entire book. I hope you were able to find value in it, and that you enjoyed the read.

As an independent author and publisher with a small marketing budget, we rely on readers, like you, to help us gain exposure with a short review on Amazon. Even leaving just a star rating, or a sentence letting us know your thoughts help tremendously!

To leave a review, [simply click here](), and you'll be taken to a page where you can give the book a rating. For those who own a physical copy of the book, it would mean so much if you did the same by visiting the product page on Amazon.

Thank you!

Thank you for your time!

Sincerely,

Michael

SOURCES & REFERENCES

Besides my own knowledge and experiences, I used the following awesome sources to create this book:

Abdur-Rahim, Yaminah. "Facial Cupping: How It Works, Benefits, Side Effects, and More." *Healthline*, Healthline Media, 1 Oct. 2018, www.healthline.com/health/facial-cupping.

Acupuncture & Massage College. "What Is Qi? Definition of Qi in Traditional Chinese Medicine." *Acupuncture and Massage College*, 28 Aug. 2017, www.amcollege.edu/blog/qi-in-traditional-chinese-medicine.

"Acupuncture, Moxa, Cupping And Herbs Relieve Asthma." *HealthCMi CEUs*, 22 July 2014, www.healthcmi.com/Acupuncture-Continuing-Education-

News/1343-acupuncture-moxa-cupping-and-herbs-relieve-asthma.

Al-Bedah, Abdullah M.N., et al. "The Medical Perspective of Cupping Therapy: Effects and Mechanisms of Action." *Journal of Traditional and Complementary Medicine*, Elsevier, 30 Apr. 2018, www.sciencedirect.com/science/article/pii/S2225411018300191.

Alban, Joseph. "Guide to Cupping for Acne - Does It Work?" *Dermveda*, www.dermveda.com/articles/cupping-for-acne.

"Allergies." *Mayo Clinic*, Mayo Foundation for Medical Education and Research, 6 Jan. 2018, www.mayoclinic.org/diseases-conditions/allergies/symptoms-causes/syc-20351497.

Ashley. "What Is Dry Cupping Therapy?" *Core Elements*, 19 Feb. 2019, www.coreelements.uk.com/2019/02/18/what-is-dry-cupping-therapy/.

"Back Pain." *Mayo Clinic*, Mayo Foundation for Medical Education and Research, 4 Aug. 2018, www.mayoclinic.org/diseases-conditions/back-pain/symptoms-causes/syc-20369906.

Berry, Jennifer. "Endorphins: Effects and How to Boost Them." *Medical News Today*, MediLexicon International, 6 Feb. 2018, www.medicalnewstoday.com/articles/320839.

Berry, Jennifer. "How to Get Rid of Bruises: 7 Effective Home Remedies." *Medical News Today*, MediLexicon International, 20 Nov. 2017, www.medicalnewstoday.com/articles/320090.

"Black Pearl Acupuncture." *Black Pearl Acupuncture RSS*, blackpearlacupuncture.com/acupuncture-pain/.

Bolen, Barbara. "Why Is My Stomach Hurting?" *Verywell Health*, Verywell Health, 29 Oct. 2019, www.verywellhealth.com/stomach-problems-causes-1945283.

Brazier, Yvette. "Wrinkles: Causes, Treatment, and Prevention." *Medical News Today*, MediLexicon International, 28 Dec. 2009, www.medicalnewstoday.com/articles/174852.

Carlotti, Paige. "What Is Cupping Therapy, and Does It Really Work?" *Men's Health*, Men's Health, 25 Feb. 2019, www.menshealth.com/health/a19519212/what-is-cupping-therapy/.

Carlotti, Paige. "What Is Cupping Therapy, and Why Does Michael Phelps Swear By It?" *Ambrosia*, 2016, www.ambrosiamassagespa.com/2016/11/13/what-is-cupping-therapy-and-why-does-michael-phelps-swear-by-it/.

Chelala, Cesar. "A Short History of Cupping." *CounterPunch.org*, 10 Aug. 2016, www.counterpunch.org/2016/08/11/a-short-history-of-cupping/.

Cherney, Valencia Higeura and Kristeen. "Tension Headaches." *Healthline*, Healthline Media, 26 Sept. 2019, www.healthline.com/health/tension-headache.

Choi, Kenneth. *Cupping Therapy for Muscles and Joints: an Easy-to-Understand Guide for Relieving Pain, Reducing Inflammation and Healing Injury*. Ulysses Press, 2018.

Conrad, Mary. *The Basics of Dry Cupping: Beginners Guide on the Benefits of Dry Cupping with Simple How-to Guide*. 2015.

Cronkleton, Emily. "How to Get Rid of Bruises: 10 Remedies." *Healthline*, Healthline Media, 8 Mar. 2019, www.healthline.com/health/how-to-get-rid-of-bruises.

"Cupping Risks / Benefits." *Cleveland Clinic*, 2017, my.clevelandclinic.org/health/treatments/16554-cupping/risks--benefits.

"Cupping, Tui Na and Moxibustion." *Blossom Wellness Centre*, 2015, www.blossomwellnesscentre.com/cupping.

Davis, Natalie Phillips and Niesha. "Ankle Pain: Causes, Home Remedies, and Prevention." *Healthline*, Healthline Media, 8 Nov. 2019, www.healthline.com/health/ankle-pain.

DerSarkissian, Carol. "Why Do My Shoulders Hurt? 13 Causes of Neck & Shoulder Pain." *WebMD*, WebMD, 25

Apr. 2019, www.webmd.com/pain-management/guide/neck-shoulder.

Ellington, Bret. "Cupping - Fire-Cupping: Healing For The Body And Mind." *Cupping - Fire-Cupping: Healing For The Body And Mind*, 2010, ezinearticles.com/?Cupping---Fire-Cupping:-Healing-For-The-Body-And-Mind&id=5578484.

"Foot Pain in Arches, Ball, Heel, Toe and Ankle Problems - Non-Injury Causes and Treatments." *WebMD*, WebMD, 14 May 2018, www.webmd.com/pain-management/guide/foot-pain-causes-and-treatments#1.

Gawne, Jennifer. "Chinese Medicine Cupping." *Chinese Medicine Cupping*, 2009, ezinearticles.com/?Chinese-Medicine-Cupping&id=2788371.

Gould, Hallie. "Does Cupping for Cellulite Work? Here's Everything You Need to Know." *Byrdie*, Byrdie, 25 Oct. 2018, www.byrdie.com/cupping-for-cellulite.

Guarneri, Mimi, et al. "Does Cupping Therapy Work? Side Effects, Benefits & Types." *MedicineNet*, MedicineNet, 12 Dec. 2019, www.medicinenet.com/cupping/article.htm.

Hecht, Marjorie. "Neck and Shoulder Pain: Causes, Remedies, Treatment, and Prevention." *Healthline*, Healthline Media, 26 Aug. 2019, www.healthline.-

com/health/what-causes-concurrent-neck-and-shoulder-pain-and-how-do-i-treat-it.

"The History of Chinese Medicine Cupping." *Kootenaycolumbiacollege.com*, 21 Aug. 2018, kootenaycolumbiacollege.com/the-history-of-chinese-medicine-cupping/.

"History of Cupping." *ACE Massage Cupping & MediCupping Bodywork Therapy*, massagecupping.com/history-of-cupping/.

Huzar, Timothy. "Does Cupping Therapy Work and What Are the Benefits?" *Medical News Today*, MediLexicon International, 29 Mar. 2019, www.medicalnewstoday.com/articles/324817.

Jadhav, Dnyaneshwar K. "Cupping Therapy: An Ancient Alternative Medicine." *Cupping Therapy: An Ancient Alternative Medicine*, 27 Mar. 2018, juniperpublishers.com/jpfmts/pdf/JPFMTS.MS.ID.555601.pdf.

Jowaheer, Roshina. "What Are Cellulite Cups and Can the at-Home Treatment Really Work?" *Prima*, Prima, 15 Jan. 2019, www.prima.co.uk/fashion-and-beauty/anti-ageing-and-skincare/a25358217/anti-cellulite-vacuum-cups/.

"Knee Pain." *Mayo Clinic*, Mayo Foundation for Medical Education and Research, 7 Mar. 2019, www.mayoclinic.org/diseases-conditions/knee-pain/symptoms-causes/syc-20350849?page=0&citems=10.

Lafayette, Amy. "The Healing Power of Cupping." *Goop*, 27 June 2018, goop.com/wellness/health/the-healing-power-of-cupping/.

"Leg Pain Causes." *Mayo Clinic*, Mayo Foundation for Medical Education and Research, 11 Jan. 2018, www.mayoclinic.org/symptoms/leg-pain/basics/causes/sym-20050784.

Malia, Michelle. "3 Questions for a Cupping Expert." *Furthermore from Equinox*, 18 Apr. 2019, furthermore.equinox.com/articles/2019/04/eqx-body-lab-cupping.

Marcin, Ashley. "What Is Cupping Therapy?" *Healthline*, Healthline Media, 4 Jan. 2019, www.healthline.com/health/cupping-therapy.

Mehta, Piyush, and Vividha Dhapte. "Cupping Therapy: A Prudent Remedy for a Plethora of Medical Ailments." *Journal of Traditional and Complementary Medicine*, Elsevier, 10 Feb. 2015, www.ncbi.nlm.nih.gov/pmc/articles/PMC4488563/.

Mehta, Piyush, and Vividha Dhapte. "Cupping Therapy: A Prudent Remedy for a Plethora of Medical Ailments." *Journal of Traditional and Complementary Medicine*, Elsevier, 10 Feb. 2015, www.sciencedirect.com/science/article/pii/S2225411014000509.

"Needling & Cupping." *Naturally Massage & Wellness*, 2016, naturally.net.au/needling-cupping/.

Nichols, Hannah. "5 Ways to Improve Skin Health." *Medical News Today*, MediLexicon International, www.medicalnewstoday.com/articles/320071.

Olson, Leslie. "Cellulite vs Stretch Marks." *PharmaQuality*, 24 May 2018, pharmaquality.com/2018/05/24/cellulite-vs-stretch-marks/.

Osborn, David K. "HIJAMA, OR CUPPING." *Greek Medicine: HIJAMA, OR CUPPING*, www.greekmedicine.net/therapies/Hijama_or_Cupping.html.

Patrik Edblad. "How to Breathe Properly - A (Surprisingly Important) Complete Guide." *Patrik Edblad*, 28 Oct. 2019, patrikedblad.com/habits/how-to-breathe/.

Peloza, John. "Causes of Lower Back Pain." *Spine*, 20 Apr. 2017, www.spine-health.com/conditions/lower-back-pain/causes-lower-back-pain.

Pietrangelo, Ann. "Why Does My Shoulder Hurt?" *Healthline*, Healthline Media, 26 Apr. 2019, www.healthline.com/health/chronic-pain/shoulder-pain.

Qureshi, Naseem Akhtar, et al. "History of Cupping (Hijama): a Narrative Review of Literature." *Journal of Integrative Medicine*, U.S. National Library of Medicine, May 2017, www.ncbi.nlm.nih.gov/pubmed/28494847.

Ratini, Melinda. "What Is Cupping Therapy? Uses, Benefits, Side Effects, and More." *WebMD*, WebMD, 2

Oct. 2018, www.webmd.com/balance/guide/cupping-therapy#1.

"Rotator Cuff Injury." *Mayo Clinic*, Mayo Foundation for Medical Education and Research, 17 May 2018, www.mayoclinic.org/diseases-conditions/rotator-cuff-injury/symptoms-causes/syc-20350225.

Rourke, Emily O. "Here's Everything You Need to Know About the At-Home Cupping Trend." *Brit + Co*, Brit + Co, 18 Nov. 2019, www.brit.co/at-home-cupping-trend/.

Tay, Melissa. "Chinese Medicine Cupping - The Process Of Cupping." *Chinese Medicine Cupping - The Process Of Cupping*, 2011, ezinearticles.com/?Chinese-Medicine-Cupping---The-Process-Of-Cupping&id=6808271.

Team, Realbuzz. "Guide To Cupping." *Realbuzz 5*, 15 Aug. 2017, www.realbuzz.com/articles-interests/health/article/guide-to-cupping/.

Team, The Healthline Editorial. "Stress and Anxiety: Causes and Management." *Healthline*, Healthline Media, 29 Sept. 2018, www.healthline.com/health/stress-and-anxiety.

"Traditional Chinese Medicine: What You Need To Know." *National Center for Complementary and Integrative Health*, U.S. Department of Health and Human Services, 29 Apr. 2019, nccih.nih.gov/health/whatiscam/chinesemed.htm.

Turner, Liraz Bergman. "Traditional Cupping Vs. Dynamic Cupping In Massage Therapy." *Heavenly Embrace Wellness in Boulder, CO*, heavenlyembrace.com/traditional-cupping-vs-dynamic-cupping-in-massage-therapy/.

Walker, Desirae. "Cupping Your Clients." *Www.massagetherapycanada.com*, 21 June 2019, www.massagetherapycanada.com/cupping-your-clients-4145/.

"Water Cupping." *Cupping Therapy*, www.cuppingtherapy.org.in/treatment/water-cupping/.

Wheeler, Tyler. "Frozen Shoulder - Symptoms, Causes, Diagnosis, Treatment." *WebMD*, WebMD, 14 Mar. 2019, www.webmd.com/a-to-z-guides/what-is-a-frozen-shoulder#1.

Wheeler, Tyler. "Shin Splints: Causes, Treatment, Recovery, and Prevention." *WebMD*, WebMD, 8 Dec. 2019, www.webmd.com/fitness-exercise/shin-splints#1.

Wheeler, Tyler. "Why Does My Elbow Hurt? 14 Common Causes of Elbow Pain." *WebMD*, WebMD, 24 Dec. 2018, www.webmd.com/pain-management/guide/elbow-pain#1.

Wong, Cathy. "Cupping Therapy Overview, Benefits, and Side Effects." *Verywell Health*, Verywell Health, 18 Jan. 2020, www.verywellhealth.com/cupping-for-pain-88933.

Made in the USA
Las Vegas, NV
21 February 2021